Nursing Practice and Education

This accessible co-produced textbook presents essential knowledge, skills, and values relevant to all undergraduate student nurses up to Master's level.

The book is structured around seven pillars of learning, which were developed through extensive consultation with patients, practitioners and academics. Each chapter focuses on an engaging scenario from nursing practice or education, which serves as the focus for the application of the seven pillars. The text is designed to meet the requirements and standards of nurse regulators internationally, including the Nursing and Midwifery Council. It includes chapters on:

- the fundamentals of nursing care
- ethics and professionalism
- evidence for practice
- patient and public involvement
- no health without mental health
- global health
- leadership and management.

The chapters include a range of features to help readers apply their learning, including the application of relevant international research and incorporating the voices of students, patients, carers and nurse educators. It enables readers to gain confidence and competence in their practice and serves as an important introduction for student nurses.

Ann Gallagher is head of health sciences and professor at Brunel University London. Ann is a registered nurse, editor-in-chief of the international journal *Nursing Ethics*, a Fulbright scholar and a fellow of the United Kingdom Royal College of Nursing. Ann's career is dedicated to progress towards excellence in health and social care through education, research and scholarship. Her most recent book is *Slow Ethics and the Art of Care* (2020). At the time of writing, Ann was head of nursing at the University of Exeter.

Kris Deering is senior lecturer and researcher in mental health nursing. Kris is lead for evidence-based practice and for mental health nursing in the Academy of Nursing at the University of Exeter. Kris has 15 years' experience in mental health nursing practice including a leadership role in a crisis team which informed his most recent book *Inter-professional Perspectives of Mental Health Crisis: For Nurses, Health, and the Helping Professions* (2022). Kris is currently researching patient-centeredness in risk management and is involved in the United Kingdom national strategy to improve risk assessment in psychiatry.

Enrico De Luca is senior lecturer and practice lead in the Academy of Nursing, University of Exeter. Enrico is a registered nurse and a qualitative/mixed methods researcher. He has an extensive clinical background in intensive care in Italy and England. Enrico's research interests include touch studies, inter-professional education, the role of spirituality in emergency, and palliative and end-of-life care. Enrico's PhD topic was mixed-method research on nurses' perceptions and education on interpersonal contact during caring. He has published research findings in international nursing journals, and his most recent publications are on the themes of palliative care in emergencies during COVID and community nursing.

Nursing Practice and Education

Aspiring to Excellence through Seven
Pillars of Learning

Edited by Ann Gallagher, Kris Deering,
and Enrico De Luca

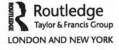
Routledge
Taylor & Francis Group

LONDON AND NEW YORK

Designed cover image: Getty Images

First published 2024
by Routledge
4 Park Square, Milton Park, Abingdon, Oxon OX14 4RN

and by Routledge
605 Third Avenue, New York, NY 10158

Routledge is an imprint of the Taylor & Francis Group, an informa business

British Library Cataloguing-in-Publication Data
A catalogue record for this book is available from the British Library

ISBN: 978-1-032-48746-5 (hbk)
ISBN: 978-1-032-48745-8 (pbk)
ISBN: 978-1-003-39056-5 (ebk)

DOI: 10.4324/9781003390565

Typeset in Sabon
by Apex CoVantage, LLC

Access the Support Material: https://www.routledge.com/Nursing-Practice-and-Education-Aspiring-to-Excellence-through-Seven-Pillars/Gallagher-Deering-Luca/p/book/9781032487458

Contents

Figures

Contributors

Howard Almond is a member of the Patient and Public Involvement (PPI) group, Academy of Nursing, University of Exeter. Howard was principal carer for his mother from 2004 till 2013 when she died with dementia at home aged 97. Diagnosed with idiopathic pulmonary fibrosis (IPF) in 2014, Howard now runs support groups for PF patients and carers in the southwest of England. He is trustee of ActionPF.org, East Teignbridge Community Transport association and Friends of Dawlish Hospital.

Nikita Bailey is a final-year student nurse on the MSci nursing programme (dual registration – adult and mental health), Academy of Nursing, University of Exeter. Nikita has a passion for caring for people in their own homes and is committed to providing dignified end of life care.

Alexander Berry is a third-year dual registration MSci nursing programme student (adult and mental health), Academy of Nursing, University of Exeter. Alex is a Sociology Graduate, Durham University and a student representative. He is interested in public health, the link between physical health and mental health and in the impact of social inequalities on health outcomes.

Marie Clancy is a senior lecturer and PPI lead, Academy of Nursing, University of Exeter. Marie is a registered children's nurse, nurse educator and researcher with special interests in creative arts based educational pedagogy and research methods. Marie's PhD research explores the experiences of children's palliative care for forced migrant families.

Susan Clompus is a senior lecturer in adult nursing and programme director for the MSci Nursing Programme, Academy of Nursing, University of Exeter. Susan's PhD study focused on resilience and paramedics from a psycho-social perspective. She has experience in realist research, service evaluation and has published in a range of nursing journals.

Patrick Coniam is associate lecturer, Academy of Nursing, University of Exeter. Patrick has a background in Medical Sciences and has worked extensively with the development and delivery of digital methods of learning and teaching in higher education. He currently teaches on topics including Anatomy and Physiology at Exeter. Patrick is also Lead for student experience and digital development within the Academy.

Isobel Coxon is a third-year MSci nursing student (dual registration – adult and mental health), Academy of Nursing, University of Exeter. Isobel is planning a career path in cardiothoracic, upper gastrointestinal and chest trauma care or community mental health. She is interested in the inter-relationship between physical health and mental health.

Kris Deering is a senior lecturer and researcher in mental health nursing. Kris is lead for evidence-based practice and for mental health nursing in the Academy of Nursing at the University of Exeter. Kris has 15 years' experience in mental health nursing practice including a leadership role in a crisis team which informed his most recent book Inter-professional Perspectives of Mental Health Crisis: For Nurses, Health, and the Helping Professions (2022). Kris is currently researching patient-centeredness in risk management and is involved in the United Kingdom national strategy to improve risk assessment in psychiatry.

Enrico De Luca is a senior lecturer and practice lead in the Academy of Nursing, University of Exeter. Enrico is a registered nurse and a qualitative/mixed methods researcher. He has an extensive clinical background in intensive care in Italy and England. Enrico's research interests include touch studies, inter-professional education, the role of spirituality in emergency, and palliative and end-of-life care. Enrico's PhD topic was mixed-method research on nurses' perceptions and education on interpersonal contact during caring. He has published research findings in international nursing journals, and his most recent publications are on the themes of palliative care in emergencies during COVID and community nursing.

Faye Doris is chair of the Patient Participation and Involvement (PPI) Advisory Group, Academy of Nursing, University of Exeter. She is a user of primary and secondary health care and has enjoyed bringing a lay voice to nurse education and the co-creation of this book.

Joel Faronbi is a lecturer and global health lead, Academy of Nursing, University of Exeter. Joel holds a doctorate degree in nursing from Obafemi Awolowo University, Ile-Ife, Nigeria. He has over twelve years' experience of mixed-methods research related to ageing. Current research interests include the health and wellbeing of older adults and their caregivers.

Ann Gallagher is head of health sciences and professor at Brunel University London. Ann is a registered nurse, editor-in-chief of the international journal *Nursing Ethics*, a Fulbright scholar and a fellow of the United Kingdom Royal College of Nursing. Ann's career is dedicated to progress towards excellence in health and social care through education, research and scholarship. Her most recent book is *Slow Ethics and the Art of Care* (2020). At the time of writing, Ann was head of nursing at the University of Exeter.

Ana Gomez Corrales is a research fellow in simulation across nursing and medical imaging teams. As an advanced neonatal nurse practitioner, Ana has experience in delivering advanced practice, acting as a role model, and promoting clinical effectiveness in care. Ana has a broad and diverse background including adult and paediatric emergency, surgical and primary care, both nationally and internationally.

Bethany Gooding is a final-year student nurse, MSci nursing programme, Academy of Nursing, University of Exeter. Beth was drawn to nursing after studying psychology and realising the connections between mind and body and the importance of care which gives each element equal importance. Beth hopes to continue underpinning her care with this philosophy when she qualifies as a dual (adult and mental health) registered nurse.

Jasmine Hesslegrave is a final-year MSci (adult) nursing student, Academy of Nursing, University of Exeter. Jasmine is interested in human and planetary health and the global health pillar. She hopes to serve as a nurse in the military, applying the global health pillar to her practice whilst treating patients in different cultural contexts in challenging clinical surroundings.

Anca Ichim is a senior lecturer and clinical skills' and simulation lead, Academy of Nursing, University of Exeter. Anca is a registered nurse whose nursing career focused on the care provided to patients requiring renal replacement therapy. Anca firmly believes that registered nurses can be inspirational leaders in every nursing intervention and is enthusiastic to be part of the MSci nursing programme, leading the clinical skills and simulation part of the nursing programme.

Matthew Jones is a second-year Mature MSci student nurse (adult and mental health), Academy of Nursing, University of Exeter. Matthew previously studied health sciences at the Open University, toured Europe as a professional musician, was a drum tutor in schools, worked with young adults and children with additional needs and managed a successful tie dye tee shirt business.

Jemima Kempton is a lecturer in nursing, Academy of Nursing, University of Exeter. Jemima is a dual registered adult & mental health nurse and has qualified in 2019. She continues to works clinically as a bank senior mental health practitioner. Jemima has research interests in professional identity, imposter syndrome and early career leadership.

Roxanne Kennedy is a final-year MSci nursing student (adult nursing), Academy of Nursing, University of Exeter. Roxanne has worked in a range of care contexts and has developed a desire to provide exceptional patient care in palliative, end-of-life, primary and community care. Interests include the field of ethics, explored further through attending conferences and co-authoring the ethics and professionalism chapter.

Richard Kyle is professor of interprofessional education in the Academy of Nursing, University of Exeter. He has diverse interdisciplinary research interests and publishes widely across nurse education and public health. Richard has held senior leadership positions in several universities, charities, and the United Kingdom National Health Service (NHS).

Mary Mancini is a member of the PPI group, Academy of Nursing, University of Exeter. Mary is from the South of Italy and moved to the UK in the year 2000. She is mother of two children. Mary is actively involved in research studies as mental health expert by experience. She worked for the NHS as an Administrator and also as a Community Interpreter.

Bel McDonald is a member of the Academy of Nursing PPI group with adult son, Fergus, who has Down's syndrome. They represent parent carers and people with learning disabilities. Bel is a parent carer, family involvement coordinator at Peninsula Childhood Disability Research unit, programme developer and lead trainer for the Healthy Parent Carers Programme.

Amy Miles is a lecturer, Academy of Nursing, University of Exeter. Amy's interests include innovative healthcare practices, compassionate leadership and service improvements which focus specifically on the integration of physical and mental healthcare. Amy is passionate about great nursing care and is excited to be part of the development of the nurses of the future.

Rachel Miller is a lecturer, research fellow and 'No Health without Mental Health' lead, Academy of Nursing, University of Exeter. As a registered mental health nurse, Rachel has experience working with veterans, military personnel, public health bodies, humanitarian organisations, and charities both nationally and internationally. Her research interests include the psychosocial implications of collective trauma, as well as inclusion health.

Leila Morgan is a lecturer, Academy of Nursing, University of Exeter. Leila is a registered nurse primarily specialising in Accident and Emergency and research. Leila has worked with trauma networks around the UK and helped deliver education to pre- and post-registration nurses. Leila's interests lie in accessible healthcare and education, trauma management and providing the best possible care for patients and their families.

Charli Morris is a final-year MSci dual registration (adult and mental health) student nurse, Academy of Nursing, University of Exeter. Charli is a member of the first cohort of this new nurse education programme. She is equality and diversity student representative and is pursuing a career path in emergency medicine and improving mental health care delivery in general hospital settings.

Oreoluwa Debs Onifade is a mental health lecturer, Academy of Nursing, University of Exeter. Oreoluwa is a registered mental health nurse in the United Kingdom and has over 22 years' experience in teaching student nurses. Currently, she is module lead for managing complexity and the academic lead for racial, equality and inclusion for the Faculty of Health and Life Sciences.

Nikole Petrova is a final-year MSci nursing student, Academy of Nursing, University of Exeter. Nikole entered the nursing world to explore her passion for health promotion and a chance to make a difference in people's lives. In addition to her core nursing interests, she aspires to experience global nursing in countries such as the United States of America.

Simon Privett is a member of the Academy of Nursing PPI group, University of Exeter. Simon is an advocate for awareness of epilepsy, and invisible disabilities more broadly. His background of lived experience has seen him deliver awareness sessions to students, clinicians, and researchers alike, bringing the lived experience perspective to those who do not have personal experience.

Lisa Reynolds is a member of the Academy of Nursing PPI group since 2020. Lisa supports the MSci nurse education programme so that a new generation of nurses practice with compassion and respect diversity, developing practical as well as inter-professional skills. She has worked as a nurse and continues in the NHS in a support role.

Hayley Rich is a final-year MSci Nursing dual registration (adult and mental health) student nurse, Academy of Nursing, University of Exeter. Hayley has an interest in emergency and trauma care and the integration of mental health care in emergency care.

Victoria Sadler is a senior lecturer, Academy of Nursing, University of Exeter. Victoria is a registered nurse with a varied career both in the UK and overseas. Her specialty in nursing and teaching is in older people's nursing with a special interest in dementia care. She works to ensure the fundamentals of care are central in all she does and to ensure people are treated with care and compassion.

Helen Smith is an administrator, Academy of Nursing, University of Exeter. Helen's contribution has been based on personal experience of dealing with a loved-one with dementia and dealing with professional organisations associated with this. This includes care homes, hospitals, primary care colleagues, community nursing, general practitioners and finally, palliative care nursing.

Holly Sugg is a lecturer/researcher in the University of Exeter's Academy of Nursing. Co-lead on the MSci nursing internship modules and previously the inaugural 'evidence-based practice' pillar lead. Research focuses on developing and testing complex interventions, specifically nursing interventions and psychological therapies for mental health difficulties, including Morita Therapy for a UK population.

Barbara Sweeney is a member of the Academy of Nursing PPI member since 2018. Barbara supports the academy of nursing so that a new generation of nurses practise with compassion and resilience, developing relational as well as transactional skills. She worked in governance and health and is currently lead governor of the local NHS Foundation Trust.

Malcolm Turner is a member of the Academy of Nursing PPI Group, University of Exeter, since 2021. Malcolm has extensive experience of health-related research as a public co-applicant and supporter of Patient and Public Involvement and Engagement (PPIE).

Welcome

As chair of the Exeter University Academy of Nursing Patient and Public Involvement Group. I have great pleasure in welcoming you to our book *Nursing Practice and Education: Aspiring to Excellence through Seven Pillars of Learning.*

I became a member of the Patient Participation and Involvement (PPI) Advisory Group in 2019. I had been put forward as a patient representative by the director of nursing in my local National Health Service Foundation Trust, where I was a public governor. I was anxious about joining this group as I had previously worked as an academic at a nearby university and this may have been seen as a conflict of interest. My fears were allayed by Nigel Reed, the then chair of the PPI group and Professor David Richards, inaugural head of nursing in the academy. Having joined the PPI group, the decision led to an active journey of involvement, co-creation, co-production, and engagement. I would even go on to say that our level of involvement was, and is, unique in nurse education programmes.

As chair of the PPI group, I feel my experience is representative of all of our members. One of our main roles has been to bring the patient's voice to the curriculum, but our involvement has been beyond that. This book is a great example of this. At the outset, the programme accredited by the nursing regulatory body, the Nursing and Midwifery Council for the United Kingdom, was based around six pillars of learning. They were: (i) fundamentals of nursing care, (ii) patient and public involvement, (iii) evidence for practice, (iv) no health without mental health, (v) leadership and management, and (vii) global health. Following the retirement of Professor David Richards and the arrival of Professor Ann Gallagher, an ethics specialist as the new head of nursing, a seventh pillar was added: (vii) ethics and professionalism. It was exciting to see the curriculum evolving.

The PPI group is now well established and is an integral part of the Academy of Nursing. We are involved in curriculum development, teaching and assessment, co-production of papers with students and academic staff, and we join the team on teaching and research days. I am proud to showcase this book as an example of fabulous co-production. Each pillar chapter, led by the pillar lead, has a PPI member in the writing team alongside a student and other teaching staff. When the PPI group was invited to collaborate on this co-produced academy book based on our pillars of learning, I must confess, it seemed like a pipe dream. We are delighted that this has now been realised and I am proud to commend this book to future students of nursing, lecturers, and nurses to keep the patient's voice at the heart of care, education, and research.

Now that I have delivered a welcome, I wish you an enriching learning experience as you work through our book. This innovative approach to education seamlessly brings together, education, research, and practice with/and the centrality of the patient's voice. I am pleased to hand over now to Professor David Richards, the Academy's inaugural Head of Nursing, who provides the foreword with more detailed background to the evolution of the seven pillars.

Faye Doris, University of Exeter

Foreword

From 2016 to 2020 I had the great honour of being inaugural head of nursing at the University of Exeter's Academy of Nursing. I led a wonderful and close-knit core team – five of us to begin with – as we developed the Academy, the first new research-intensive UK university nursing school in the 21st century. We were advised by a huge cast of patient and carer colleagues, local clinical directors of nursing, practicing nurses, experienced nurse educators, student guild and university senior academic and professional services representatives, joined soon after by our first lecturers and clinical lecturers. (I do not have permission to include individuals' names here, but you know who you are and how much the core development team and I appreciated your varied, expert, and extensive input.)

As a development team, we were all convinced that we really had to offer something radically different. So the first thing we did was eliminate 'modules', those small self-contained educational units which are ubiquitous in education and which students tick off as they amass sufficient academic credits to qualify as a nurse. Why did we do that?

In our view, modules artificially divide course content. I was once told by a Norwegian nurse educator and researcher that when third-year nurses attended her courses they were 'lost to her'. She wanted them to use research in their practice, but it was too late for them. They had completed that module, 'ticked the box' and moved on. Research, like many other subjects, was just one more module to be studied, exams passed, and then ignored.

So, rather than modules, we developed the pillars that are the subject of this book. We wanted our pillars to represent the essential elements of nursing practice, to be incorporated into every single lesson, constantly reinforced and reiterated, to be woven into the teaching and learning fabric of our courses.

But what should these pillars be? We consulted our patient, carer and senior nursing colleagues on our options. But I confess that here it also did get personal – you see, I have skin in the game. As well as being a nurse, I have been a patient. I have experienced both fabulous nursing care and frank neglect. Once, having negotiated my way through three separate triage systems, I sat in agony with a dangerous and spreading infection and overheard a charge nurse describe me as an 'inappropriate referral'. I have been looked after expertly by caring and skilled nurses and I have also lain immobile in a hospital bed without assistance to wash and toilet myself. I have seen variations in practice between those based on tradition and ritual and those driven by the best evidence. I have, at first hand, witnessed staggering health disparities in which 80% of children with cancer in low to medium income countries die, whilst 80% of their compatriots in high income countries survive. I have seen nurses spend time listening to people in great mental distress and I have seen other nurses scuttle away from such conversations for fear of where they will lead. I have worked with both inspirational leaders and managers who were mostly absent.

Our team of educators, patients, carers, clinicians, and senior leaders found that we all shared similar experiences. So, choosing the pillars was easy. They fell straight out of our lived experience of nursing, as practitioners, patients, carers and scientists. We did debate them of course. Our patient and carer colleagues were particularly forthright about fundamental nursing care, researchers were equally adamant about nursing science, and senior nurses advocated for strong leadership. But, eventually, we all agreed that we were on exactly the right track with our choices.

If asked, I could not in all honesty say which pillar is the most important. For sure, our most recent Exeter research programme on fundamental nursing care, including both the developmental 'ESSENCE' project and then one of the largest randomised controlled trials of nursing care globally – 'COVID-NURSE' – meant that fundamental care was up there without question. I am also a mental health nurse and psychotherapist who rages at the inequity and stigma inherent in the way we spilt education between physical and mental health. That was not going to happen on my watch.

From my very first days as a student nurse, I have sought out opportunities to hear from patients and members of the public about their own experiences of health, illness, and care. I cannot abide health systems designed for the convenience of those that work in them rather than those that use them (pretty much every single health system I have come across to be brutally frank). We listened carefully as our patient and carer colleagues told us about their experiences. As a team, we also wanted to ensure that newly qualified nurses could read, use and produce solid scientific evidence for what they do; to value evidence and to understand how science can contribute to enhanced experiences of care for those we look after. Unlike my Norwegian colleague, we did not want any of our Exeter nurses to be 'lost to us'.

In an era of increasing nationalism, we also wanted our nurses to look beyond their borders, to reach out past our shores. We wanted them to see that health transcends geographical and economic barriers. How ironic, then, that as our first nurses began their educational journey in Exeter, we saw the starkest reminder of this truth as the COVID-19 pandemic swept across the world, leaving no corner untouched.

Finally, and something that was very dear to the hearts of our senior nurse colleagues, we wanted our nurses to inspire others. To be able to lead and manage teams with courage and conviction. To provide guidance, support, and care to those they work with. We wanted the Exeter Nurse to be someone others could look up to; a name that would resonate around the world as a mark of excellence, leadership and competence.

So there they were, our pillars: fundamentals of care; no health without mental health: patient, patient and public involvement, evidence for practice; global health; leadership and management. At the time we missed one out. However, the second academy head of nursing, Ann Gallagher, included ethics and professionalism as a seventh pillar. This committed the Exeter nurse to professional values including social justice, compassion, dignity, and integrity, and to the flourishing of individuals, families, and communities. I could not agree more.

I hope this book will help you embed these essential seven principles in your teaching, research, and practice. If you are a patient or someone's care partner, I especially wish you experience the best care that these pillars represent. We really believe they will drive nursing care through the 21st century and beyond. Good luck with using, receiving, and teaching the pillars.

David A. Richards, Bergen, Norway

1 Introduction

Ann Gallagher, Kris Deering, and Enrico De Luca

Introduction

This is an exciting time to be a nurse. A time when nurses have never been more needed to respond to local and global health challenges. A time for nurses to assume leadership opportunities to manage increasing care complexity. A time for nurses to promote social justice by enacting advocacy – and allyship – with all those in need of fundamental care. And a time to recognise the value – and necessity – of continuous professional learning which contributes to excellence in health and social care.

Nursing is a moral and relational practice, requiring engagement in relationships with patients, families, communities, colleagues, technology and the environment. Nurses appreciate repeated recognition as the most trusted profession (Royal College of Nursing, 2022a). During and after the COVID-19 pandemic, there was recognition of nurses' significant contributions to patient and family care through a most difficult period (International Council of Nurses, 2021b).

Globally, there are critical staff shortages in health and social care. The International Council of Nurses (2021a) estimate that there will be a future global shortfall of 13 million nurses. The United Kingdom (UK) National Health Service (NHS) is described as being in 'crisis', with shortage of nurses, fewer graduates, and 48% of nurses joining the UK Nursing and Midwifery Council register coming from overseas (Royal College of Nursing, 2022b). Intense debate exists regarding professional migration, as registered nurses travel to the UK and other higher income countries from lower income nations, with calls for ethical recruitment from the International Council of Nurses (2019). Nurses have a critical role in recovery and rebuilding the profession (International Council of Nurses, 2023) and in stepping up to fill gaps in local provision.

Career opportunities for nurses continue to develop and evolve, embracing a wide range of roles in care practices. This includes roles as practitioners, leaders, educators, and researchers as well as evolving roles in digital health, sustainability, genomics, patient safety and public health. The pandemic shifted nurses' attention from the local to the global, underscoring the value and importance of solidarity with nurses in other cultural contexts. Reflection on expertise and experience necessary for a contemporary professional, in ever-changing times, becomes more pressing. This book demonstrates that necessary nurses' knowledge, skills and values are captured by the seven pillars of learning, as introduced in the chapters that follow, namely: fundamentals of nursing care; ethics and professionalism; evidence for practice; patient and public involvement; no health without mental health; global health; and leadership and management.

DOI: 10.4324/9781003390565-1

The development of the seven pillars, as outlined in the foreword by professor David Richards, inaugural head of nursing at Exeter, aligned with the creation of a new and innovative nurse education programme. As the book demonstrates, the pillars of learning have wide and international application. The pillars were co-created with patients, carers, clinicians and researchers and act as golden threads throughout nursing practice and nurse education. A commitment to the pillars will contribute to student nurses' preparation for nurse leadership, to the aspiration to promote and strive for excellence in health and social care and to being the best they can be as registered nurses and leaders.

The co-production of this book has been an inspiring and affirming collaborative process at a time of great local, regional, and global challenges. We take the view that co-production is a process of democratic enquiry in the creation of something of value for all involved parties. Hence, those traditionally seen to hold expertise, such as nurses, require awareness of the imbalance of power and work towards all views being worthy of equal attention. Co-production aims to challenge asymmetrical power, associated with the traditional expertise of health professionals, and work towards the collaborative generation of knowledge in relation to nursing practice and education and which is, importantly, meaningful to those directly impacted such as patients and their families (Norton, 2022).

This introductory chapter explores four core themes, comprising the acronym CARE, which are integral to the ethos of this book and in accord with the seven pillars: curiosity; advocacy; respect; and excellence. Each theme will be explored in turn and revisited in the concluding chapter. Thereafter, an outline of each chapter will be provided, particularly surrounding their purpose. First, we turn to curiosity.

Curiosity

In the text *How Humans Learn: The Science and Stories Behind Effective College Teaching*, Joshua E. Eyler (2018) points to 'patterns' which contribute to learning and which are drawn from multidisciplinary research. The five patterns are: curiosity, sociality, emotion, authenticity, and failure. Whilst all of these are interesting and relevant to the learning journeys of students and practitioners, curiosity is arguably the first and foremost element in progression towards excellence in nursing practice and education. Curiosity is a necessary prerequisite to engagement with, and understanding of, the seven pillars of learning.

So, what is curiosity? Why is it necessary? And how does it manifest in nurse education and practice?

Eyler (2018) cites a definition of curiosity from Emily M. Grossnickle (2016, p. 26): 'At its core, curiosity is the desire for new knowledge, information, experiences or stimulation to resolve gaps or experience the unknown.' Acknowledging gaps requires the ability to be reflective and to demonstrate an open mindedness regarding the impossibility of knowing everything. This is to inspire the pursuit of knowledge, building confidence and awareness in how to ask questions and appreciate the areas of knowledge needed to progress towards excellence in professional life.

In his writing about 'purposeful curiosity', Costas Andriopoulos (2022, pp. 5–6) explains why curiosity matters:

Curiosity has long been the driving force of survival and progress. Across evolutionary time, curious animals were more likely to survive because they understood and adapted to their environment. Throughout history, humans crossed borders and pushed into new territories to find a better place to live, to make a fortune, or simply to discover what was on the other side . . . Embracing purposeful curiosity allows us to discover whole new worlds. Without risks and the discomfort of newness there can be no creative or intellectual breakthroughs. Curiosity is how we evolve, stretch ourselves, and make connections that and discoveries that not only enrich our own lives but can change the world.

Andriopoulos (2022, p. 7) provides guidance as to how we might benefit from curiosity. First, he explains that we need to have 'the right mindset'. By this, he means making time and space to think. This aligns with the scholarship of one of the editors regarding 'slow ethics' (Gallagher, 2020, pp. 75–96). It is important to feel comfortable with one's own thoughts and, for example, walk slowly in nature, take tea and reduce external stimuli, to develop connection and understanding of the self, and one's thoughts. The third recommendation regarding mindset, is to 'activate a sense of wonder' (Andriopoulos, 2022, pp. 9–10). This reminds us to nurture a sense of awe and wonder, going beyond our professional and disciplinary contexts, to better appreciate the complexity and beauty of our environment and care ecosystem. This includes attention to, and appreciation of, the composition, capabilities, and shortcomings of humans, other species, and the environment. Such attentiveness requires effective questioning to develop understanding, alongside awareness of the types of knowledge necessary to progress our field.

Eyler (2018, p. 43) writes that 'each academic field can be *defined* by its essential questions'. If we allow that nursing is an academic field, as well as a professional field, we need to discuss which essential questions define our field? Might perspectives on nurses' patterns of knowing guide our questions? That is, questioning can be contingent on contexts, such as clinical setting, treatment and underlying philosophies, and all these can inform the notion of patterns.

In 1978, Barbara Carper published the seminal paper around 'fundamental patterns of knowing in nursing'. Carper identified four patterns of knowing: empirical (drawn from research evidence), personal (from critical reflection on own values and purpose), ethical (descriptive and prescriptive ethics) and aesthetic (knowing related to the art of nursing) (Cody, 2013). Since, other patterns of knowing have been identified, namely, emancipatory knowing, socio-political knowing and spiritual knowing (Lindell and Chinn, 2022). Each pattern of knowing is associated with critical questions which provide a direction of travel in suggesting essential questions that define nursing.

Before turning to *advocacy*, a note about knowledge and humility. The concept of 'cultural humility' is referred to in the patient and public involvement pillar chapter of this book (Chapter 5). It is an important consideration for reflection on diverse care contexts. Reflection on a broader sense of humility is helpful as we exercise curiosity in our practice as nurses, leaders, educators and researchers. This enables us to balance pride in our practice with the awareness that we are limited in rationality, sympathy and knowledge. De Vries (2019) refers to this perspective from Mayeroff (1971, p. 25):

> Pride in a job well done is not pretentious, it does not distance; rather it goes with an honest awareness of what I have done and the extent of my dependence on the co-operation of others and on various conditions. There is nothing incompatible between pride, in this sense, and humility.

As mentioned above, the co-production of this book, which included members of our patient and public involvement group, student nurses and members of the nurse education team, stimulated our creativity and enabled a balancing of pride in our achievement with humility. None of us has all the answers and it was recognised that there is much to gain from listening and inviting feedback. The process also emphasised the importance of advocacy and the adoption of a critical approach to a much discussed concept in the nursing literature. In advance of the discussion in Chapter 9, we introduce a complementary concept – allyship – alongside advocacy, in the next section.

Advocacy

It is now 50 years since advocacy made its appearance in the nursing literature, with the recommendation in the 1973 International Council of Nurses Code that nurses should advocate for patients. Section 1.7 of the current Code states: 'Nurses advocate for equity and social justice in resource allocation, access to health care and other social and economic services' (International Council of Nurses, 2021c). Section 3.4 of the NMC Code (Nursing and Midwifery Council, 2018) states that nurses should 'Act as an advocate for the vulnerable, challenging poor practice and discriminatory attitudes and behaviour relating to their care.'

Discussions of advocacy remind that, in addition to representing the rights and interests of patients, nurses also advocate for communities, for policy change, for individual nurses/themselves and for the profession (Dworak-Peck, 2017). However, there is a caveat. In recognition of the asymmetrical power that nurses can hold, advocacy, in its truest sense, might seem tokenistic. Advocacy means also recognising when nurses are unable to help, for example, when associated with legislation to confine patients in mental health contexts. For nurses to accept that, in some instances, they may be unable to help due to legal obligations, requires broad-mindedness as to who is better placed to help. Hence, advocacy also involves bringing in neutral parties that can, more authentically, advocate for the patient voice (Water et al., 2016). A systematic review regarding 'nurses' perspectives of patient advocacy' (Saleh et al., 2020) proposes that preparing nurses for the role of patient advocate is essential. It also concluded that the concept, as noted above, is complex, used variously and should be considered a process with four components: 'the patient situation, the nurse, the advocacy action, and the advocacy care outcome' (Saleh et al., 2020).

A concept which has appeared recently, and is complementary to advocacy, is that of allyship. Guidance from the United States, in the context of activism against domestic and sexual violence (Oregon Coalition Against Domestic and Sexual Violence, undated, p. 1), suggests a working definition of allyship as:

> an active, consistent, and arduous practice of unlearning and re-evaluating, in which a person holding systemic power seeks to end oppressions in solidarity with a group of people who are systematically disempowered. Since everyone holds systemic power in some areas and lacks it in others, everyone has areas in which they can practice allyship.

Activities to enact allyship include listening, respecting lived experience (and expertise gained through experience), providing solidarity unconditionally, stand beside people, respect their history, learn to articulate how oppressive systems work, prepare to make mistakes and apologise (see Oregon Coalition Against Domestic and Sexual Violence, undated). Regarding differences between the 'ally', 'advocate', and 'activist', Ragazzo (2020) states:

To be an ally is to support. To be an advocate is to amplify problems occurring in society. To be an activist is to take intentional action to bring about change, typically social or political. Society can't move forward without them.

Throughout the process of producing this book, we were reminded repeatedly, and helpfully, of the value of meaningful participation and sharing of perspectives. The involvement of patients, carers and students in, for example, the development of scenarios and application of the pillars, proved to be enriching. Whilst the theme of nurse advocacy ran through most of the scenarios, the theme of allyship permeated the production process. It is our hope that student nurses, who read our book, will recognise the opportunity and imperative to take a stand, becoming activists in relation to equity, social justice and the climate crisis.

A spirit of mutual respect characterised our engagement with each other, underpinning the theme of the next section.

Respect

'Respect' appears on many organisational lists of values and is integral to professional codes, however, it is rarely explained. Many years ago, one of the editors (AG) published a paper on the theme of 'The Respectful Nurse' (Gallagher, 2007). The paper opened with a sign at London Zoo's small animals' enclosure: 'Shhh . . . Please respect the animals by walking quietly' (p. 360). Rarely is there such clear behavioural guidance regarding how we might enact respect in the human care context.

The concept of 'respect' is usually heard or read as a directive urging 'respect', in relation to other humans, species and the environment. The concept is also utilised in relation to values which are central to nursing practice and to the seven pillars discussed in this text. You will read, for example of respect for autonomy, respect for human rights, respect for dignity, respect for privacy, respect for confidentiality and respect for persons. In relation to each of these ethical imperatives, there is the opportunity and need to reflect on their meaning and implications. In general terms, each indicate actions and ways of thinking on the part of students, registered nurses, and educators, in relation to each of the seven pillars of learning.

The process of co-production of this book was underpinned by a commitment to learn from diverse perspectives of members of our patient and public involvement (PPI) group, from students and from members of the nurse education team. Our regular book development meetings enabled general discussions feeding into chapter team meetings. All required respect and, at times, compromise as we worked together to agree roles, responsibilities and deadlines. This was in the spirit of authentic co-production, with academic authors required to relinquish power to ensure the views of all involved contributed to the production of the chapters.

Excellence

One of the discussions, during the co-production of this book, related to the title. Some were committed to the title 'Excellence in nursing practice and education . . .', while others questioned if such attainment was possible within an ever-evolving world? and what this implied about our humility if we were to make such a claim? A PPI group member – Simon – suggested a way forward. The title should indicate an aspiration, a pursuit embedded with hopefulness to do and be the best we can and to continuously aspire to betterment. We are indebted to Simon, therefore, for stimulating a consensus that our book title should include the words 'aspiring to excellence'.

The concepts of 'excellence' and 'aspiration' capture the essence of what we, as authors, consider the overall message of this book. Excellence in health and social care is what we aspire to and what student and registered nurses should aim towards. Excellence is the end aspired to and involves a receptiveness to engaging with past scholarship and to the development of new knowledge, contributing to ever-evolving care practices. But nurses also need to reflect on what 'excellence' means in relation to their professional practice, in their relationships with patients, families and communities, in relationships with members of multi-professional teams and with technology and the environment. Nurses also need to reflect on the meaning of excellence' in relation to their roles as nurse practitioners, leaders, educators and researchers.

Pat Riley, who is described as one of the greatest basketball coaches and as a 'masterful motivator' (Geoffreys, 2018, p. 96), proposed: 'Excellence is the gradual result of always striving to do better.' The idea of excellence as the end of a process which aims to do (and be) better is persuasive. The idea of each of us as 'works in progress' is helpful as we consider diverse learning journeys and reflect on our fallibility and imperfection. The learning journey from student nurse to registered practitioner and beyond is captured through the seminal text by nurse academic, Professor Patricia Benner, *From Novice to Expert: Excellence and Power in Clinical Nursing Practice*. Benner (2001) combines empirical research with the Dreyfus model of skills' development (Dreyfus and Dreyfus, 1980). The model details five levels of proficiency as: novice, advanced beginner, competent, proficient, and expert. Benner (2001) illuminates each of these levels with qualitative research with 'beginning' and 'experienced' nurses. There is insufficient space to do justice to Benner's work here, however, an extract from the preface relates her approach to excellence in nursing (Benner, 2001, p. xxi):

> descriptive research that identified five levels of competency in clinical nursing practice. These levels – novice, advanced beginner, competent, proficient and expert – are described in the words of nurses who were interviewed and observed either individually or in small groups. Only patient care situations where the nurse made a positive difference in the patient's outcome are included. These situations offer vivid examples of excellence in actual nursing practice.

The detail of the care situations illuminates the features of the different levels of practice and suggests the importance of student nurses learning from observations of, and engagement with (see Chapter 9), peers and registered nurses in practice. Insights regarding excellence and leadership – what all of us 'should' aspire to – intersect with many professions and areas of practice. Florence Nightingale reminds us that nurse leaders have obligations beyond their own behaviour, and that they play an important role in sustaining ethical cultures of care: 'how can I provide for this right thing always to be done?' (Nightingale, 2010 [1859]).

One area of practice, closely aligned with nursing in its earlier years, is the military. A recent text titled *The Habit of Excellence: Why British Army Leadership Works* (2021, p. 244) by Lieutenant Colonel Langley Sharp MBE provides the following conclusion, which serves as a fitting end to this section:

Good leaders have a bias to action and a tendency to reflection. They lean on tradition and experience, without ever losing sight of what is around them and ahead of them. Most importantly, they recognise that the individual who continues to learn is the one who will continue to lead, inspiring trust and belief in those who follow them. Every leader, of whatever age and role, remains a lifelong work in progress. For those curious and humble enough to seek them out, the most important lessons always lie ahead.

The next section provides a summary of the chapters in this book relating to the seven pillars of learning, commencing with an illustration (Figure 1.1) summarising each pillar.

The Chapters

Each of the chapters, which focuses on a specific pillar, has a similar format. The chapters detail anonymised scenarios, an introduction to the pillar and application of the pillar to the scenario. Each chapter conclude with 'takeaways', that is, with summary points for students and for educators and practitioners, to capture key points made in the chapter.

Chapter 2: The Fundamentals of Nursing Care Pillar

The chapter engages with the experience of 39-year-old Jay, diagnosed with pulmonary fibrosis, and explores the care received in an intensive care unit. Nursing is experiencing wide-ranging changes, with technology, increasingly complex care interventions and research developments contributing to improvements in outcomes. However, the art of nursing exemplified in fundamentals of care, is necessary to complement – and enhance – intensive care technological interventions. Hence, this chapter reminds that attention to holistic assessment and person-centred communication, to reducing environmental stressors and to eating, drinking and comfort are as essential as technological and pharmaceutical interventions.

Chapter 3: The Ethics and Professionalism Pillar

The chapter focuses on a scenario relating to the residential care experience of Mrs Brenda McCarthy, who lives with dementia. The chapter introduces approaches to ethical theory which are applicable to nursing. These include approaches based on duties, rights, consequences, and virtues. The well-known principles of biomedical ethics (although not favoured by all nurse ethicists) are a helpful and accessible approach to the analysis of care scenarios, particularly when combined with a virtue-based approach. The ETHICS deliberative framework is applied to the scenario, illustrating, among others, the value of approaching ethical aspects of care situations in a systematic manner.

Chapter 4: The Evidence for Nursing Practice Pillar

The chapter introduces evidence-based practice in relation to a 21-year-old student, Onisha, who experiences mental distress within an emergency department. The chapter sets out what can be meant by evidence but also takes a particular position, that evidence needs to be led, not only by professional expertise, and sources such as research, but also patient views. Corresponding to pragmatist philosophy, evidence can also be perspective driven, with relevance to particular times and places. There is also critique of absolutes in the vein of pragmatism, around the best ways to produce research with the study aim, not necessarily the methodology, informing the research design.

Chapter 5: The Patient and Public Involvement Pillar

The focus of this chapter is the care of 10-year-old refugee Naajy and his family. Naajy has a life-limiting condition, however, rather than focus on limitations, his strengths are utilised to enhance his care. Naajy and his family are involved in nurse education, illustrating the importance of PPI. The scenario and analysis stimulate reflection on the importance of cultural humility and on creative strategies to involve patients, family and the public in nurse education, care and research. Nurses need to demonstrate commitment to respectful, authentic participation of patients, families and the public in nurse education. They need also to take a stand to end tokenistic approaches, thus creating opportunities to increase creative and meaningful engagement.

Chapter 6: The No Health without Mental Health Pillar

The chapter engages with the complexity and interrelationship between physical and mental health regarding 41-year-old Matthew, who is experiencing mental distress owing to several social stressors. Emphasis will be on seeing health, not as the absence of mental health, but as intricately integrated with physical health within our lives. Nevertheless, there remains a disparity with seeing mental health as important to other health factors. Hence, the chapter examines Mathew's experience and demonstrates the necessary interrelationship between physical and mental health, working towards holistic models of care that consider the whole person. Equal consideration for mental and physical health also enhances patients' ability to embrace a personal sense of recovery.

Chapter 7: The Global Health Pillar

Focusing on the experience of registered nurse, Titi, this chapter introduces global aspects of health and nurse migration. Titi has migrated from Nigeria to the UK and works in an infectious diseases' care context. Global health includes recognition of the impact of the climate emergency, poverty and inequalities on health. This is an emerging field, particularly in its application to nursing. The chapter draws on the scenario to provide an overview of some of the most significant issues that impact on health within a global context, alongside implications for nurse education and practice. Given that the field has grown substantially, in relation to nursing, in the 21st century (Leffers *et al.,* 2017), the chapter urges a shift in nurses' focus from the local to the global, to think beyond borders and to consider health in terms of citizenship of the world.

Chapter 8: The Leadership and Management Pillar

The chapter introduces leadership and management with a scenario drawn from a nurse education context. It concerns simulation lead Melanie providing support to lecturers George and Mia, who recently transitioned from clinical practice to roles in a university. The chapter provides opportunities to reflect on distinctions between management and leadership and on a range of leadership theories. Leadership roles are assumed by student and registered nurses as they, for example, role model good practice, provide support to colleagues and inspire others to aspire to excellence. Insights gained from critical engagement with the scenario and theories introduced, can be applied to leadership and management roles in numerous contexts. These include leading education teams, supporting the development of fellow students in practice or on campus, coordinating shifts on a hospital ward and being the lead investigator on a research project.

Chapter 9: Integrating the Seven Pillars of Learning

This penultimate chapter, authored by students, brings together insights from the seven pillars in relation to the experience of student nurses, Rachel and Ashley, as they work with Fatima in a palliative care context. The uniqueness of this chapter is that the voices of students have priority, providing a lens into their world as they apply the seven pillars of learning to the care of Fatima and negotiating student relationships. The discussion includes analysis of the fundamentals of nursing care pillar, acknowledgement of the place of ethics and professionalism, the role of evidence, global health in relation to cancer and consideration of mental and physical health Moreover, the uniqueness of Fatima and breaking down of barriers to embrace authentic participation is addressed in terms of PPI, with attention also to student well-being and to cultural and gender diversity. Lastly, the leadership and management pillar discussion focuses students' reflection on peer support, role modelling and allyship.

Chapter 10: Conclusion

The final chapter returns to the opening CARE themes of curiosity, advocacy, respect, and excellence in relation to the seven pillars and wide range of related topic areas explored in the previous nine chapters. Providing opportunities for readers to take stock of learning as they journey through the book, reflective questions are included for student self-assessment with suggestions for educators to stimulate critical reflection as they utilise the text. The last chapter, therefore, aims to inspire learners and educators as they aspire – together – to excellence in health and social care.

Conclusion

It is not usual, or recommended, to add new content to a conclusion. However, we concluded that the previous discussion implies a question which should be reflected on as readers engage with this text: What makes a good nurse?

Related to this are questions related to what supports or undermines the practices of nursing and education. Nurse and philosopher Derek Sellman (2011, p. 20) writes: 'Nursing, like teaching, contends with a number of internal and external pressures, some of which have the potential to undermine basic assumptions about the practice itself.' As readers journey through our co-produced book, we invite reflection on additional critical questions implied by this quotation: What are the internal and external pressures that undermine the practice of nursing? How should nurse leaders respond to these pressures? And why does the continuation – and strengthening – of nursing as a discrete profession, and as an art and science, matter?

It is hoped that the pillars of learning represented throughout the book will resonate with readers and strengthen their commitment to develop and advance the profession. It is hoped, too, that readers will recognise their critical role in supporting the flourishing of patients, families, and communities. We hope, finally, that confidence

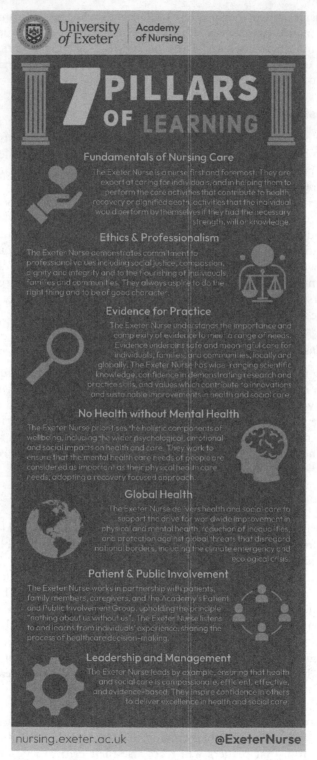

Figure 1.1 Outline of the seven pillars of learning

and competence gained from working through this book and availing of numerous learning opportunities will retain focus on the aspiration to excellence in health and social care.

A Note on Terminology

We recognise the existence of different terminology relating to those who receive care, support, and a wide range of interventions from nurses and other health and social care professionals. Terminology includes, for example, 'client', 'resident', service user', and 'survivor' in different care contexts. However, in this book, we generally refer to 'patient' as this the term is recognised globally and, whilst the term can be disputed, we mean this to be inclusive and as encompassing alternative terminology as above.

References

Andriopoulos, C. (2022) *Purposeful Curiosity: How Asking the Right Questions Will Change Your Life*. London: Yellow Kite.

Benner, P. (2001) *From Novice to Expert: Excellence and Power in Clinical Nursing Practice. Commemorative Edition*. London: Prentice-Hall International (first edition 1984).

Carper, B. (1978) 'Fundamental patterns of nursing', *Advances in Nursing Science*, 1(1), pp. 13–24 (republished in W.K. Cody (ed.), *Philosophical and Theoretical Perspectives for Advanced Nursing Practice*, 5th edition, London: Burlington. Jones and Bartlett Learning, 2023, pp. 23–33).

Cody, W.K. (2013) Values-based practice and evidenced-based care: Pursuing fundamental questions in nursing philosophy and theory. In W.K. Cody (ed.), *Philosophical and Theoretical Perspectives for Advanced Nursing Practice*, 5th ed. Burlington, MA: Jones and Bartlett, pp. 5–14.

Dreyfus, S.E. and Dreyfus, H.L. (1980) *A Five-Stage Model of the Mental Activities Involved in Directed Skill Acquisition*. Unpublished report supported by the Air Force Office of Scientific Research (AFSC) USAF (Contract F49620-79-C-0063). Berkeley CA: University of California at Berkeley.

Dworak-Peck, S. (2017) '5 ways nurse practitioners can serve as advocates'. Available at: https://nursing.usc.edu/blog/5-ways-nurse-practitioners-can-serve-as-advocates/ (Accessed: 19 April 2023).

De Vries, K. (2019) 'Humility and helplessness in the realization of limitations within hospice'. In J. Cole Wright (ed.), *Humility*. New York: Oxford University Press, pp. 227–249.

Eyler, J.R. (2018) *How Humans Learn: The Science and Stories Behind Effective College Teaching*. Morgantown, WV: West Virginia University Press.

Gallagher, A. (2007) 'The respectful nurse', *Nursing Ethics*, 14(3), pp. 360–371.

Gallagher, A. (2020) *Slow Ethics and the Art of Care*. London: Emerald Publishing.

Geoffreys, C. (2018) *Pat Riley: The Inspiring Life and Leadership Lessons of one of Basketball's Greatest Coaches*. Florida: Calvintir Books.

Grossnickle, E.M. (2016) 'Disentangling curiosity: Dimensions, definitions, and distinctions from interest in educational contexts', *Educational Psychology Review*, 28(1), pp. 23–60.

International Council of Nurses. (2019) 'International Council of Nurses calls for ethical recruitment to address critical shortage of nurses'. Available at: www.icn.ch/news/international-council-nurses-calls-ethical-recruitment-process-address-critical-shortage (Accessed: 23 April 2023).

International Council of Nurses. (2021a) *ICN Policy Brief: The Global Nursing shortage and Nurse Retention*. Geneva: International Council of Nurses.

International Council of Nurses. (2021b) 'The COVID-19 effect: World's nurses facing mass trauma, an immediate danger to the profession and future of our health systems'. Available at: www.icn.ch/news/covid-19-effect-worlds-nurses-facing-mass-trauma-immediate-danger-profession-and-future-our (Accessed 23 April 2023).

International Council of Nurses. (2021c) 'The ICN code of ethics for nurses'. Available at: www.icn.ch/node/1401 (Accessed 23 April 2023).

International Council of Nurses. (2023) 'Recover to rebuild: Investing in the nursing workforce for health system effectiveness'. Available at: www.icn.ch/publications/recover-rebuild (Accessed 23 April 2023).

Leffers, J., Levy, R.M., Nicholas, P.K., and Sweeney, C.F. (2017) 'Mandate for the nursing profession to address climate change through nursing education', *Journal of Nursing Scholarship*, 49(6), pp. 679–687.

Lindell, D. and Chinn, P. (2022) 'Overview – patterns of knowing in nursing'. Available at: https://nursology.net/patterns-of-knowing-in-nursing/ (Accessed 23 April 2023).

Mayeroff, M. (1971) *On Caring*. Translated by Alphonso Lingus. London: Harper and Row.

Nightingale, F. (2010 [1859]) *Notes on Nursing: What It Is, and What It Is Not*. Cambridge: Cambridge University Press.

Norton, M.J. (2022) 'Co-production and mental health service provision: A protocol for a scoping review', *BMJ Open*, 12(5), pp 1–5.

Nursing and Midwifery Council (2018) 'The code: Professional standards of practice and behaviour for nurses, midwives and nursing associates'. Available at: www.nmc.org.uk/standards/code/ (Accessed 23 April 2023).

Oregon Coalition Against Domestic and Sexual Violence (undated) 'The handout'. Available at: https://vawnet.org/material/working-definition-allyship-handout (Accessed 19 April 2023).

Ragazzo (2020) Ally, Advocate and Activist: Understanding Who We Are in the World Demanding Change. Available at www.linkedin.com/pulse/ally-advocate-activist-understanding-who-we-world-honorio-ragazzo (Accessed: 24 April 2023).

Royal College of Nursing (2022a) 'Nursing confirmed as "most trusted profession" as strike risk grows'. Available at: www.rcn.org.uk/news-and-events/Press-Releases/nursing-confirmed-as-most-trusted-profession-as-strike-risk-grows (Accessed: 23 April 2023).

Royal College of Nursing (2022b) 'Investing in patient safety outcomes'. Available at: www.rcn.org.uk/Professional-Development/publications/investing-in-patient-safety-and-outcomes-uk-pub-010-567 (Accessed: 23 April 2023).

Saleh, U., Aboshayga, A., O'Connor, T., Saleh, M., Patton, D. and May, A. (2020) 'Nurses' Perspective of Patient advocacy: A systematic mixed studies review', *International Journal of Nursing and Clinical Practices*, 7. Available at: www.graphyonline.com/archives/IJNCP/2020/IJNCP-317/ (Accessed: 23 April 2023).

Sellman, D. (2011) *What Makes a Good Nurse?* London: Jessica Kingsley Publishers.

Sharp, L. (2022) *The Habit of Excellence: Why British Army Leadership Works*. Dublin: Penguin Random House.

Water, T., Ford, K., Spence, D. and Rasmussen, S. (2016) 'Patient advocacy by nurses – past, present and future', *Contemporary Nurse*, 52(6), pp. 696–709.

2 The Fundamentals of Nursing Care Pillar

Enrico De Luca, Victoria Sadler, Alexander Berry, Isobel Coxon, and Howard Almond

Introduction

Fundamentals of care (FOC) is, quite deliberately, the first pillar of learning discussed in this book. The pillar underpins the core ethos of the Academy of Nursing and signals the priorities of the founder members and commitment of the current team. The pillar engages with a movement, a framework, and an aspiration to reclaim a vision of nursing which is care-focused, collaborative, person-centred, and relational.

In June 2012, a group of nurse leaders, researchers, clinicians, and policy experts came together at Green Templeton College, University of Oxford, to debate and agree an action plan to integrate FOC with the person-centred care (PCC) agenda (Kitson et al., 2013). The group recognised that, while there has been progress in the delivery of patient-centred care, there continue to be challenges in 'meeting the basic needs of many of our most vulnerable patients due to a range of complex factors' (Kitson et al., 2013, p. 2). The meeting resulted in the development of a framework, an action plan and, later, an international network of those committed to fundamentals of care in response to the needs of patients, families and communities. Patient needs are met by developing positive and trusting relationships with the care-recipient as well as their family and carers (Feo et al., 2017).

Introducing the anonymised scenario of a patient, Jay, who requires nursing care in an intensive care unit (ICU), we explore the fundamental elements of care needed. This ranges from the accuracy of vital signs' recording to the safety requirements of medicine administration and to the care of someone who needs support with their hygiene and elimination needs. This also includes the compassionate communication skills required when supporting patients and their families. This chapter draws on scholarship and re-search relating to FOC, maintaining the focus on nurses' essential skills, knowledge, and values.

The criteria for ICU admission include patients at risk of deterioration who require urgent closer monitoring of physiological variables through invasive and non-invasive means, providing support for a single (or more) failing organ system. Intensive care units also deliver enhanced post-operative care (Stretch and Shepherd, 2021). We apply elements of the FOC framework, which ensures, in all care contexts, continuity of care, patient-centredness, a holistic approach, enhanced communication skills, and the use of interpersonal contact within caring relationships (Minton et al., 2018).

DOI: 10.4324/9781003390565-2

Scenario

Jay is a 39-year-old male, recently diagnosed with pulmonary fibrosis. This is a lung disease involving scarring of the lung tissue, which results in reduced gas transfer between the lungs and the blood.

Jay has a partner, Laura, and two children, Olivia (aged twelve) and James (aged nine). Jay has a large network of friends as he used to play in a local football team. He enjoyed his work as a car mechanic but recently, due to his respiratory condition, he had to take sick leave from the garage.

In the last weeks, following an episode of flu, Jay experienced a deterioration in his physical health. Although Jay is usually able to manage his respiratory crisis with small periods on oxygen therapy, delivered via a portable oxygen concentrator, he was struggling to breathe. Laura called an ambulance and Jay was taken to the emergency department of the local hospital. After a few hours of observation and assessment, Jay was transferred to ICU.

Following admission to ICU, Jay was assigned to Anna, a very experienced ICU nurse. Anna fully monitored his condition, took blood samples, performed a physical assessment, and started to outline an integrated nursing care plan. Jay needed assistance to change positions, with personal hygiene, and to feel comfortable. His anxiety further impeded his breathing, and he was prescribed medication (a mild anxiolytic) to reduce agitation. Anna prioritised strategies to reduce local stimuli (sounds, alarms, volume settings etc.) to help Jay relax and focus only on his breathing. In addition, Jay was experiencing pain when coughing, which increased his physical and emotional distress.

After a few hours in ICU, Jay experienced haemodynamic instability. Haemodynamic instability can be defined as perfusion failure, represented by clinical features of circulatory shock and advanced heart failure (Vincent and De Backer, 2013). He also had a high temperature (39°C), reduced saturation of oxygen (85%) and difficulty with breathing. Anna reported to the ICU anaesthetists this sudden deterioration of Jay's conditions, while also explaining the management plan to Jay. This would consist of non-invasive ventilation but also a possible intubation if Jay's health deteriorated further.

Jay asked why intubation was needed, in terms of the consequences of the procedure and possible alternatives. Anna and the ICU team explained to Jay that endotracheal intubation – for invasive ventilation – would rarely be used for a patient with pulmonary fibrosis, as it could lead to further exacerbation of the condition. Nevertheless, this is considered an emergency intervention. During the conversation Jay also asked if Laura can be involved with making this decision, or at least be informed. He requested that his family be contacted so they can be with him.

Jay's general health was deteriorating fast, as indicated also by arterial blood gas exchange. Anna took an arterial blood sample from Jay and performed the analysis. Arterial blood gas analysis provides information on oxygenation as well as information on the respiratory status of the person (Castro et al., 2022). Anna explained to Jay the need to start non-invasive ventilation (NIV) to ensure Jay could make an informed decision about the treatment, while also reassuring him. Non-invasive ventilation is delivered via specific ventilators using a facial or nasal mask, with or without oxygen. Non-invasive ventilation delivers differing air pressure depending on inspiration and expiration. It is considered a good compromise for patients with pulmonary fibrosis because the procedure can help to avoid intubation during respiratory crisis (Moran et al., 2017).

The NIV special mask and the high airflow made communication difficult, and Jay was becoming more anxious. Anna supported him by ensuring that his family was present, and, with Jay's consent, they were kept informed of Jay's condition. As well as the non-invasive ventilation, it was determined that Jay needed antibiotics and steroids to treat an infection that was also impeding his breathing.

The respiratory crisis was resolved within 24 hours, and the NIV was reduced, with use of antibiotics continuing as prescribed. Jay remained in ICU for another day and was then sent to the respiratory ward and went home two days later.

Fundamentals of Care: What Are They?

The original FOC group (Kitson et al., 2013) agreed that any working definition should include aspects of Virginia Henderson's description of the 'unique function of the nurse':

> To assist the individual, sick or well, in the performance of those activities contributing to health or its recovery (or to peaceful death) that he would perform unaided if he had the necessary strength, will or knowledge.
>
> (Henderson, 1964, p. 15)

To many patients, the nurse is the constant feature of their care experience, especially in a healthcare setting. Nurses can have a profound impact on people's lives, often being able to form therapeutic relationships with the person and their wider family (Burton and Ludwig, 2014; International Council of Nurses, 2021). It is the nurse who supports someone to meet their physical needs when they are unable to be independent. It is the nurse who provides emotional and psychological support, and it is often the nurse who seeks to understand and guide a person through their health and social care needs (Burton and Ludwig, 2014).

The need for care, and the delivery of that care, are key parts of the nurse-patient relationship. Central to this are fundamentals of care (Mudd et al., 2020). All too often the care activities of supporting hygiene, nutrition and elimination are described as 'basic nursing care', overlooking the complex interrelations of these activities and missing the fundamental right that people have to expect this care, when they are unwell (Ryder et al., 2021; Kitson et al., 2014).

A danger of perceiving these nursing interventions as 'basic' is that they can become viewed as less valuable or less important to learn about or provide. Unfortunately, the downgrading of FOC practices, can lead to patients potentially receiving poor care as widely reported in recent years (Feo et al., 2019; Feo and Kitson, 2016; Kitson et al., 2014). Global failures in health and social care often feature inattention to personal hygiene needs, lack of emotional support to patients and families and missed opportunities for communication and dignity. These, and many more examples of care deficits, can result from the devaluing of fundamental care practices (Feo and Kitson, 2016).

In considering the reasons why we, as nurses, may under-utilise FOC practices, it appears that the reasons are varied. There is, perhaps, pressure on services, an increased level of multi-morbidities to respond to and the sense that people, especially in acute hospital settings, are experiencing high acuity and complex needs (Feo and Kitson, 2016). The effect of managerial structures, performance indicators and dominance of the medical model can also be seen as potential reasons for the downgrading of the fundamentals of care (Feo and Kitson, 2016).

However, we also need to acknowledge that nursing as a profession has potentially allowed this move away from fundamental care. Meeting hygiene needs, eating and drinking may all be seen as self-care skills. Most people when well, and not experiencing mental or physical health deficits, can perform these activities themselves. As people become unwell, they may no longer be able to meet these needs and do need assistance. Traditionally, this has been the role of the nurse. However, some nurses may value technical skills more and see the fundamentals of care as elements of practice delivered by non-nurses (Feo and Kitson, 2016). Nurses may, for example, delegate this care to care-assistants or auxiliary staff and student nurses on placements which may indicate that such care as less valued. Students may come to value technical skills, completed by registered staff, over relational and fundamental care, believing that the learning of the latter is not required or of less value (Feo and Kitson, 2016; Feo et al., 2018, 2019). To ensure that patients are assisted to meet their needs when unable to do so, the nursing profession needs to lead and revalue fundamental care practices.

A Framework for the Fundamentals of Care

Debate and discussion at Templeton Green College, referred to in the introduction, resulted in the initial FOC framework with three core dimensions:

> statements about the nature of the relationships between the nurse and the patient within the care encounter; the way the nurse and the patient negotiate and integrate the actual meeting of the fundamentals of care; and the system requirements that are needed to support the forming of the relationships and the safe delivery of the fundamentals of care.
>
> (Kitson et al., 2013, p. 2)

The 2012 meeting led to the development of the International Learning Collaborative (ILC), an organisation involving nurse academics and researchers, dedicated to ensuring that the FOC are visible and valued in every care setting globally. The ILC aims to influence care settings worldwide refocusing attention on the FOC, recognising the challenges that may affect them, while seeking ways to overcome these challenges (Kitson et al., 2019). International Learning Collaborative members designed the Fundamentals of Care framework (Figure 2.1) to outline how care should be in any health and social care setting and for any care recipient to receive care in an effective, safe, and high-quality manner:

> The framework comprises of a series of concentric circles that integrate the core relational elements at the centre with the outer system requirements at the periphery. Central to the framework is the relationship between the patient and the nurse.

This relationship is based on a commitment by the nurse to care for the patient (and significant others). The nurse also has a commitment to communicate the information about the patient to other staff, relevant carers, and family members. This ensures consistency and continuity of care as the patient moves from dependency to independence in self-care activities (or indeed, continues to be dependent on others).

(Kitson et al., 2013, p. 12)

The framework outlines three core dimensions for the delivery of high-quality fundamental care (Kitson et al., 2013):

1. **The relationship**. A trusting therapeutic relationship between care recipient and care provider.
2. **Integration of care**. Integrating and meeting the persons' needs to create individualised care plans. Nurses will consider needs surrounding the physical (safety, warm, clean, fed, dressed, comfortable and pain free, rested, mobile and hydrated), psychosocial (supporting coping mechanisms, self-care, providing a calm environment, give respect, understanding and dignity) and relational (involvement with decision making, respected and supported).
3. **The context of care**. Nurses involved with leadership, resourcing, staffing, and broader policy and regulatory issues that influence the quality of the nurse-patient relationship. This includes exploring the impact on the nurse-patient relationship in terms of the wider healthcare system, settings and/or contexts.

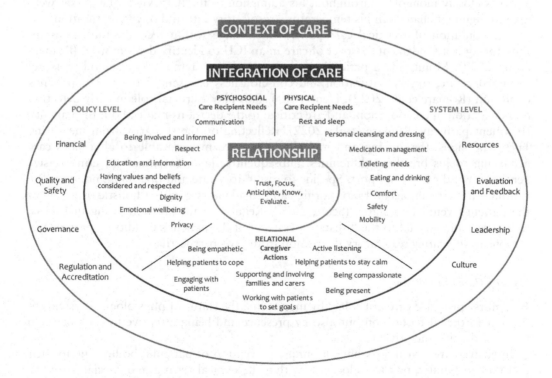

Figure 2.1 The fundamentals of care framework

Image obtained from https://ilccare.org/the-framework; content within image derived from Feo et al. (2017)

The framework relies upon nurses' ability to connect with the patient and through that connection be able to meet, or help, the patient to attain their fundamental care needs (Kitson et al., 2013). The overall focus is on enabling the patient and the nurse to assess confidently and competently and to plan, implement and evaluate care integrating fundamental care needs. In addition, the framework describes person-centred care trajectories. It does not, therefore, focus directly on therapeutic aims or diagnosis but on the facilitation and coordination of care.

Application of Fundamentals of Nursing Care Pillar to Scenario

Despite ICUs being renowned as high-tech and fast-paced environments, the following discussion explores how FOC addresses the care needs of Jay and his family. This demonstrates how FOC is an inherent part of ICU nursing practices. Alongside continuous monitoring and management of infusions, detecting and preventing complications, use of ventilators and management of other devices, nursing in ICU manifests features of care that we argue are fundamental. By doing so, we show how such practices form an integral part of ICU nursing. We focus on the following aspects of care: monitoring vital functions; nursing care of the body; holistic assessment; comfort rounds; communication skills; minimising environmental stressors; health literacy in critical care; and ethical challenges.

Monitoring Vital Functions

Jay was closely monitored throughout his admission to the ICU where the nurses were able to highlight changes in his temperature, respiratory rate and oxygen saturations.

The condition of a critical care patient can change within seconds; thus, constant monitoring is a fundamental aspect of care in an ICU to identify deterioration (Romare et al., 2022). Monitoring a patient's vital signs including temperature, blood pressure, respiratory rate, oxygen saturation and consciousness is essential to track a patient's condition (Romare et al., 2022). Hence, vital signs play a crucial role in early detection and escalation of deterioration, and are critical to the decisions made about the patient's treatment pathway (Romare et al., 2022). Reflecting on the scenario, from measuring Jay's vital signs, the nursing and multidisciplinary team were able to alter Jay's care according to his breathing difficulties. Subsequently, Jay was placed on non-invasive ventilation and oxygen support. Specific to respiratory rate and breathing, non-invasive ventilation interventions and monitoring can provide nurses with a holistic overview of the patient's ventilation status (Scott, 2019). Regular vital sign monitoring in ICU is, therefore, fundamental to the holistic assessment of the patient's condition, particularly symptoms indicating respiratory depression from Jay's perspective.

Nursing Care of the Body

Jay's nurse provided care not solely by monitoring the status of physiological systems to prevent further deterioration but also by presence and being attentive to Jay's needs in terms of dignity and privacy.

Intensive care unit nurses have a unique perception of patients' bodies due to their constant proximity, physical closeness within the clinical setting and special access to the personal intimacy of patients (Benner, 2002). The reflections about intimacy barriers are often taken for granted by nurses (and by other health professions too). This has inspired a corpus of studies on the importance of physical dimensions which, ideally, are embodied as part of nursing care (Draper, 2014). ICU nurses have many occasions to provide care through the bed bath, touch, infection and pressure sores prevention, eye, and mouth care, providing comfort, and changing the patient's position while in bed (Karlsson et al., 2022).

Bringing back the focus to FOC can help ICU nurses to realign with a vision of the patient's body as less objectified, and in harmony with the unspoken signals from the patient, representing subtle changes with their health needs (Lawton and Shepherd, 2019). Yet, nurses may struggle with such delicate practices given the depersonalised nature of medicine, in that they remain neutral to make objective decisions. Hence, it is important to be attuned to a style of caring which respects the person's biography and individuality. This develops a social connectedness that mitigates indifference seen with the detachment of the medical model, despite the patient being sedated and unable to communicate (Roulin and Spirig, 2006; De Luca et al., 2021).

Holistic Assessment

Alongside capturing objective health-related data, Jay's nurse also enquires about Jay's history and other details he feels are meaningful, while also gaining such data from his family.

Intensive care unit nurses assess patients, adopting a systematic approach to observe every physiological system and develop a nursing care plan to meet specific needs at any time (Jakimowicz and Perry, 2015). This process implies not only observing objective data, elicited by the continuous full monitoring of machinery, but also all the subjective data gathered from the proximity and access to Jay's body (such as chest auscultations, observing chest movements, skin integrity status, bowel movements and nutrition status). Although ICU nursing for some might be grounded in the biomedical 'cure-oriented' approach, maintaining patient-centred nursing is based on the physical wellbeing of the patient, including fundamental elements of psychological and social care. Gaining a holistic patient history ensures Jay is known as a person with a life beyond the ICU and not just a clinical entity. When the person is awake, ICU nurses are not just obligated to take a history but also crucial is collaborating (and extending care) with families, and any significant others. Hence, all aspects of the person are considered, incorporating a biopsychosocial model, as to humanise Jay's care as much as possible (Lehman et al., 2017). This will be further explored in the' no health without mental health chapter' (Chapter 6).

Comfort Rounds

In the ICU, Jay was nursed in bed and required assistance with positional changes. However, this was more than just moving the patient and included understanding as to why such positional changes, among other care approaches, were needed.

Evidence plays a vital role in all aspects of nursing and it is essential for all student and registered nurses, to keep abreast of the latest evidence that informs their area of practice (Youngblut and Brooten, 2001). In terms of the fundamentals of nursing care, evidence is recognised as integral to providing the best possible care for patients (Nelson, 2014). The primary reason for comfort rounds is to change Jay's position in bed and prevent the formation of pressure ulcers by checking the skin for deterioration. However, comfort itself is also a significant factor, and through changing positions, Jay may feel the attention is calming, while also feeling less isolated. When in ICU, a conscious patient may be experiencing fears about their mortality. Moreover, changing Jay's position is a good time to check if his needs are being attended to such as promoting hydration and dignity, for example, ensuring Jay is not exposed. Comfort rounds are a frequent intervention and essentially provide opportunities to enrich the consistency of FOC practices, by nurses interacting with patients if conscious and ensuring comfort for those unable to communicate (Carby et al., 2017).

Communication Skills

With the scenario, the nurse communicated with Jay and ascertained he was experiencing anxiety and pain while coughing.

Communication plays a vital role in the delivery of FOC practices, and can involve adoption of different techniques to communicate, especially when the patient is intubated. Nurses need to ensure the person is understood (using a communication board for example, whereby patients point to letters, words, or pictures). Communication with sedated patients is a sensitive practice. As nurses, we need to listen and look to any signs from the patient, such as heart or respiratory rate during manoeuvres, or any little twitching or muscular activity.

Communication is more than just the ability to have a conversation, it also requires understanding what the patient is experiencing as well as how the person expresses concerns (Kourkouta, 2014). With such communication, nurses are able to gain information and advocate for patient needs, not only with providing high-quality care, but also to prepare a meaningful care plan shaped by the patient views (Bramhall, 2014). Communication, however, goes beyond the patient-nurse relationships, extending also to family members. In environments such as the ICU, it can often be fast paced, and patient conditions may rapidly change, hence, important to keep family members updated so they feel included and reassured. Moreover, communication with family members is critical to avoid providing fragmented information which can also ensure that the family are receiving adequate support (Adams et al., 2017).

Minimising Environmental Stressors

The noise and discomfort caused by NIV, in terms of noise, airflow and the fitted mask, and inability of Jay to remove himself from the disturbances may add unnecessary stress.

Intensive care nurses have a duty to reduce environmental stressors (involving noises and lighting) that may induce post-ICU syndrome or mental distress, especially once the patient's health improves, and the person is preparing for discharge. Post-ICU syndrome refers to physical, cognitive, and mental impairments that occur during an ICU stay, after ICU discharge, or hospital discharge. This can also influence the long-term prognosis of ICU survivors (Inohue et al., 2019). Nurses have opportunities to supervise this crucial phase of the patient's recovery and to propose measured interventions, which reduce the impact of environmental stressors. Gezginci et al. (2022) suggested that environmental stressors may trigger emotional changes of the patients (whether anxiety, depression, and/or anger), determining the effectiveness of the treatment and hospitalisation process. Hence, FOC involves ICU nurses with the vital role of identifying and reducing environmental stressors, alongside teaching patients how to mitigate the impact of such disturbances.

Health Literacy in Critical Care

With Jay's consent, his family were kept informed about his condition and treatment and also the significance of the devices, alarms and monitors. This helps orientate the family to the ICU setting.

A common source of distress for family members is receiving complex and fragmented information by the ICU medical team (Young et al., 2017). There may be a language barrier, due to cultural differences (as explored in Chapter 5), but also language barriers with the use of medical jargon, when updating the family (Ingram and Kautz, 2012). Family members who receive proactive meetings with the distribution of understandable information tend to experience less post-traumatic stress, anxiety and depression compared to control groups (Young et al., 2017). To that end, Jay's nurse explained to his family the plan for care, alongside the care process and the workings of the equipment using accessible language and practical examples. The FOC framework includes explanations and inclusion of family members so they can participate in care, with a view to enhancing the patient's recovery. Thus, any nursing intervention in ICU requires exploration of the health literacy of the family to shape meaningful communication, while regularly checking that all information provided is understood (Yeh and Ostini, 2020).

Ethical Challenges

Jay's nurse informed Jay and his family of the benefits and risks of intubation so an informed decision can be made about the recommended treatment.

Nursing in ICU means exposure and involvement with ethical challenges. The ethics and professionalism chapter explores ethical challenges in care further (Chapter 3), Jay and his family have the right to be involved in decision-making, necessitating access to current information (Fernandes and Moreira, 2013). There is strong evidence and obligations to be inclusive when making treatment decisions. This requires the inclusion of voices, which are significant within the patient's life, especially when the patient lacks a voice and there are no safeguarding concerns (Luce, 2010).

An ethical obligation implies a nursing role of patient advocacy, so the patient's rights to self-determination. This might include weighing up the best interests of the patient when there is a lack of consensus (Flannery et al., 2016). To discuss such similar topics in more depth, the chapter now turns to the use of reflection and its abilities to ground nurses within FOC to ensure the optimum care for patients. Please see Chapter 3 for discussion of other ethical perspectives.

An Approach to Reflections on the Scenario

To ensure nursing is embedded within FOC practices, reflection is a crucial part of the act of caring to contemplate what approaches work well and what might be improved. To that end, the following is an example of such reflection, adopted to consider the care provided by Jay's ICU nurse. This is not only to highlight the value of reflection, but also, to underline that reflection is a pivotal part of FOC, ensuring that care is meaningful and beneficial to patients.

It is important to recognise that reflective practices come in different forms and tend to draw on the philosophy of John Dewey (1933) who advocated a methodical approach and the scholarship of Donald Schön (1983, 1987). Schön cites the importance of intuitive knowledge in responding to situations. While the reflective model outlined below denotes a frequently adopted method, leaning towards the views of Dewey (1933), the reflection is also informed by Schön in terms of learning from the engagement in and on action.

Reflective practices also embrace clinical supervision, which involves discussing a clinical situation either individually with a supervisor or in a group setting (Hawkins and Schwenk, 2011). The purpose is to learn from dialogue with another/others. Some approaches adopt a counsellor viewpoint whereby the supervisee reflects introspectively about personal past events that influence current circumstances (Hawkins and Schwenk, 2011). Restorative supervision, for example, is widely adopted within healthcare (Wallbank, 2013). It is solution-focused, drawing on the A-EQUIP model, which is 'advocating for education and quality improvement', hence, supervisees are guided to learn from their experiences, with allowance for catharsis around difficult situations. Emphasis is placed on considering solutions (Lister, 2022).

Although reflection is advocated in the chapter, and throughout the book, it is not without criticism. It has been argued, for example, that the use of models can constrain creativity by following a linear pathway, which is not how all situations arise or how learning necessarily occurs (Seaman, 2008). Individual reflection can also be limiting, given the process of self-evaluation and the likelihood that we will not know all our inner thoughts nor realise all that is needed to challenge ourselves (Greenwood, 1993). Alternatively, reading and inviting feedback regarding our responses from patients, for example, help to develop a comprehensive care repertoire (Schön, 1983). This ultimately is what we advocate in the reflection below which suggests the nursing perspective in reflecting on caring for Jay. This summarises important considerations around FOC practices. Underlying this are themes discussed in Chapter 1, particularly in relation to the role of curiosity and humility. That is, there is always more to know about ourselves and situations around us, including when care is incorrectly assumed as 'basic'.

The 'What' Model of Reflection

The following discussion is underpinned by the principles of reflection in- and on- action, as developed by Schön (1983). To reflect-in-action we need to consider the situation and act immediately to make any relevant changes to our approach, such as how we can mitigate challenges and consider what we should do or say in the situation (Schön, 1983). Alternatively, reflecting on, or after the action, enables consideration of the experience from a distance, to understand what we may value from the experience and explore what we may do differently in future. Importantly, we need to identify why we may make changes or continue with the same approach (Schön, 1983).

Anna, in the chapter's scenario, is constantly reflecting in her practice. Anna will know what she is doing in the provision of Jay's care and has built professional knowledge and expertise to be able to provide high standards of nursing (Schön, 1983). Anna has self-belief that she can provide fundamentals of care, while also knowing what she is doing, evolving her practice to meet Jay's individual needs. Anna's reflection in-action allows her to be prepared to meet challenges, to react to changes in Jay's condition, be prepared to meet his care needs and be in readiness for the unexpected (Schön, 1983).

As a continuous reflector, Anna will need to reflect after the experiences, to explore any immediate insights and consider in retrospect what she may do differently or the same when faced with similar events. Reflecting after action allows practitioners to consider the experience in retrospect, to draw on different perspectives as illustrated above, and gain a deeper understanding of their experiences (Williams, Wooliams, and Spiro, 2020).

In the scenario, Jay has a respiratory condition that does not always require ICU intervention and may potentially mean that Anna has not cared for someone with pulmonary fibrosis. Anna can draw on her experience of caring for other people requiring respiratory support in ICU. After her experience with caring for Jay, Anna should ideally reflect on this situation, to continue to develop and build her skills, and this can be enabled by reflecting after action (Schön, 1983).

The use of a reflective model enables a structured approach to our reflections. Nurses can use a model to analyse and understand their experiences, to build their knowledge and nursing skills (Williams et al., 2020). In this chapter, we have focused on the FOC, hence, we are going to use a reflective model to reflect on Anna's actions when providing care for Jay.

The model allows us to reflect on an experience by asking:

- **What?** What occurred and what is the focus of the reflection;
- **So what?** What is the meaningfulness to the nurse in terms of the situation; and
- **Now what?** What actions such as learning considerations and nursing practices in case such a situation reoccurs (Driscoll, 2007).

Using this model, we can explore the scenario while the subsequent learning can inform and develop our practice. We have chosen to reflect on Anna's ability to meet the FOC as Jay's condition deteriorated. As an experienced nurse, Anna may choose to reflect on her knowledge specifically related to pulmonary fibrosis. Anna may identify that she met Jay's needs well, that she fulfilled his FOCs while also identifying his deteriorating condition and her suitable responses. However, Anna may acknowledge that she has not encountered people with pulmonary fibrosis before and so may want to focus her learning on aiding people with the condition.

What?

Jay has been admitted to ICU due to a deterioration of his pulmonary fibrosis. He is supported by Anna who is experienced, not just with the highly technical environment of ICU, but also in the delivery of the fundamentals of care. Even in the highly technical setting of ICU, it is important that the needs of the person are met, there is provision of person-centred care, and indeed, that the FOC are adopted. Anna may be completing complex tasks but also has a duty to humanise the care provided to Jay.

Jay is restricted in his abilities to meet his own fundamental care needs. As an experienced nurse, Anna should be able to identify what Jay can do, supporting Jay with completing these needs as he feels empowered. She also acts as a substitute to provide needs that Jay cannot complete (Cuzco et al., 2021). From the scenario, we see that Anna assists Jay with personal hygiene, ensuring his privacy and dignity is maintained. Anna also supports Jay with regularly changing his position to avoid complications associated with prolonged bed rest, notably pressure ulcers. Moreover, Anna completes vital signs and interprets the recordings, so Jay receives the correct treatment at the right time. Such monitoring is constant, to observe for changes in Jay's condition and act accordingly, as well as swiftly, on this information (Romare et al., 2022).

In the scenario, we see the vital importance of communication with Jay and his family, highlighting communication as fundamental to his care. This contributes to building a therapeutic relationship between Jay and Anna, the nurse.

The following quotation comes from Howard Almond (co-author and patient and public involvement representative). He is living with pulmonary fibrosis and has had experience of being in hospital in several different environments:

> It is very important to listen to the patient and his family, to understand the build-up to the crisis and nature of the underlying problems. In this case, continuing oxygen therapy will be required into the future, and it is possible that this episode will have caused progression in the underlying pulmonary fibrosis. While progression is possible, it is not a foregone conclusion so it is important for the team to reassure the patient and his family that monitoring will continue to establish what, if any, long-term effects there will be.
>
> (Howard, PPI group member)

So What?

The person-centred care that Anna is providing for Jay is central to the FOC and to everything she is doing (Belle et al., 2020). Of course, it is important that, as an experienced ICU nurse, Anna is recognising the signs of Jay's deterioration, that she is responding to changes in his haemodynamic status, responding to the changes in his oxygen requirements and working with the ICU multi-professional team to stabilise Jay's physical condition. These are all critical care skills required to maintain Jay's health and support him with an evidence-based scientific approach. Furthermore, Anna has recognised that Jay is not able to care for himself, given his critical condition, and requires support to meet the care activities that normally he can achieve himself, notably washing, dressing, moving, and eating (Feo and Kitson, 2016; Kitson et al., 2014). Anna also ensures that there is a clear line of communication between Jay, his family and the other professionals in the ICU to provide coherent updates and limit the fragmentation of information.

In this chapter, we have acknowledged that, sometimes, it is nurses themselves who see FOC practices as less important or valued than the technical skills, perhaps, seeing such practices as 'basic' and for auxiliary staff (Feo et al., 2018, 2019). However, we also see that Anna in the scenario is performing both the technical skills and the fundamentals of Jay's care, ensuring his needs are met when he is unable to do so. Nurses like Anna who value the FOC challenge task-orientated care and, instead, prioritises patient-centeredness. Jay is considered a whole person with biopsychosocial needs. He is regarded as more than a patient with a condition that merely requires treatment (Belle et al., 2020; Feo and Kitson, 2016).

If we look at the FOC framework, in relation to Anna's approach to Jay's care, we can see she is not only meeting his physical needs but also the psychosocial and relational elements which contribute to the integration of care (Belle et al., 2020; Feo et al., 2018). As Anna focuses on Jay's comfort – reducing environmental distractions and through the support to change his position – Anna is addressing the psychosocial elements of keeping Jay calm and addressing physical elements of safety, warmth, rest and comfort (Feo et al., 2017; Kitson et al., 2014). The care Anna delivers is empathetic and respectful as to build a therapeutic relationship with Jay (Feo et al., 2017; Kitson et al., 2014).

The integration of care dimension of the FOC framework, focuses on the assessment of persons' needs, encouraging carers to recognise their factors of independence and dependence (Feo et al., 2017). Anna may support Jay with some of his physical care needs when he may be less independent. However, by keeping Jay informed, explaining and supporting his understanding of the plans for his care, Anna is maintaining his independence, enabling Jay to make informed choices about his care plan, while also involving his family with such decision-making.

Anna's actions, as she supports and provides care for Jay, allows her to work within the first dimension of the framework: the relationship (Feo et al., 2017). We see Anna able to focus on Jay, understanding and interpreting his needs, building and maintaining a trust. We also see that through her communication with Jay and his wife, Laura, Anna seeks out their opinions, so they feel valued and feel some control in a challenging situation.

Now What?

As we have explored in this chapter, the FOC can easily be eroded and lost. This can be due to many factors such as service pressure or focusing on managerial or medical frameworks. Or, as we discussed above, nurses who undervalue FOC practices and downplay their importance (Feo and Kitson, 2016). In this chapter, we have argued that nurses – in every setting – need to commit to and promote the fundamentals of care. Mindful of the substantial literature that emphasises human needs, for example, Maslow's hierarchy of needs (Maslow, 1954), it is clear that nurses' commitment to FOC is a necessary response to the range and complexity of these needs.

Conclusion

This chapter demonstrates how fundamentals of care are needed in every clinical setting, including in the intensive care unit. The scenario, relating to Jay's care and treatment, enables reflection on the complexity of care and caring relationships when confronted with the high demands of technological nursing and care responses in emergencies. Intensive care unit nurses occupy a special position in nursing with an impressive body of knowledge, skills and clinical expertise. Integrating the fundamentals of care with more technical clinical care, in diverse care contexts, provides opportunities to revalue elements of nursing, retaining the focus on the person at the centre of care.

The role of nurses, as proposed by Virginia Henderson (1964), remains relevant to contemporary nursing. Nurses need to value and prioritise fundamentals of care which enable them to assist individuals with activities that contribute to enhancing health, recovery or to a peaceful death. As demonstrated in the application of FOC to the care of Jay and his family, nurses' contribution to improving the condition and experience of patients is significant. This is the case whether patients are in ICU, in the community or in any other care context. Their contribution enriches quality of life and honours the commitment to care, proposed by Virginia Henderson and proponents of the fundamentals of care framework.

Takeaways for Student Nurses

- A student nurse should avoid describing care as 'basic'. The FOC framework reminds us that care is complex, valued, impactful, and anything but basic.
- Observations of care experiences enables you to reflect on episodes where you have seen the FOC applied. Detail the elements of the FOC framework you witness and compare with learning from this chapter.
- Take opportunities to identify nurses who prioritise elements of FOC in their practice and consider how you might emulate their practice.
- Describe and apply critical thinking to a scenario where nurses seem unaware of the FOC. Reflect on how you might be a change agent in such situations and role model FOC in your practice.
- As a student nurse and an individual, you can inspire others to prioritise FOC practices. Consider how you can support the confidence and competence of other students in this area.

Takeaways for educators/practitioners

- The FOC realigns nursing with the importance of caring relationships and the value of nursing with authenticity and person-centred care.
- Teaching, fostering, and supporting the FOC in nurse education help students to embrace a humanistic paradigm and bring back invaluable care concepts into clinical settings.
- Encouraging students' interest in the FOC challenges students' perceptions of 'basic care' and enables them to recognise their significant contribution to holistic care.
- The FOC framework provides specific lenses and tools to guide nurses in assessing and safeguarding in clinically complex settings.
- Educators and practitioners must ensure that students perceive their responsibility to advance FOC and appreciate the privilege of nurses' contribution to excellence in health and social care.

References

Adams, A., Mannix, T., and Harrington, A. (2017) 'Nurses' communication with families in the intensive care unit – a literature review', *Nursing in Critical Care*, 22(2), pp. 70–80.
Belle, E., Giesen, J., Conroy, T., van Mierlo, M., Vermeulen, H., Huisman-de Waal, G. and Heinen, M. (2020) 'Exploring person-centred fundamental nursing care in hospital wards: A multi-site ethnography', *Journal of Clinical Nursing*, 29(11–12), pp. 1933–1944.
Benner, P. (2002) 'Caring for the silent patient', *American Journal of Critical Care*, 11(5), pp. 480–481.
Bramhall, E. (2014) 'Effective communication skills in nursing practice', *Nursing Standard*, 29(14), pp. 53–59.
Burton, M. and Ludwig, L. (2014) *Fundamentals of Nursing Care: Concepts, Connections and Skills.* Philadelphia: F. A. Davis Company.

Carby, J., Davis, R. and Ashley, R. (2017) 'Comfort rounds: task-orientated nursing or effective care?', *BMJ Supportive and Palliative Care*, 7(Suppl 2), pp. A70–A71.

Castro, D., Patil, SM. and Keenaghan, M.(2022) 'Arterial blood gas'. Available at: https://europepmc.org/article/NBK/nbk536919 (Accessed: 12 April 2023).

Cuzco, C., Torres-Castro, R., Torralba, Y., Manzanares, I., Muñoz-Rey, P., Romero-García, M., Martínez-Momblan, M.A., Martínez-Estalella, G., Delgado-Hito, P. and Castro, P. (2021) 'Nursing interventions for patient empowerment during intensive care unit discharge: a systematic review', *International Journal of Environmental Research and Public Health*, 18(21), pp. 11049–11063.

De Luca, E., Fatigante, M., Zucchermaglio, C. and Alby, F. (2021) 'Awareness to touch: A qualitative study of nurses' perceptions of interpersonal professional contact after an experiential training', *Nurse Education in Practice*, 56, pp. 1–8.

Dewey, J. (1933) *How We Think: A Restatement of the Relation of Reflective Thinking to the Educative Process*. Chicago: Henry Regnery.

Draper, J. (2014) 'Embodied practice: rediscovering the 'heart' of nursing', *Journal of Advanced Nursing*, 70(10), pp. 2235–2244.

Driscoll, J. J. (2007) 'Supported reflective learning: the essence of clinical supervision?' In J. J. Driscoll (ed.), *Practising Clinical Supervision: A Reflective Approach for Healthcare Professionals*. London: Bailliere Tindall, pp. 27–52.

Feo, R. and Kitson, A. (2016) 'Promoting patient-centred fundamental care in acute healthcare settings', *International Journal of Nursing Studies*, 57, pp. 1–11.

Feo, R., Conroy, T., Jangland, E., Athlin, A., Broval, M., Parr, J., Blomberg, K. and Kitson, A. (2017) 'Towards a standardised definition for Fundamental care: A modified Delphi study', *Journal of Clinical Nursing*, 27, pp. 2285–2299.

Feo, R., Donnelly, F., Frensham, L., Conroy, T. and Kitson, A. (2018) 'Embedding fundamental care in the pre-registration curriculum: Results from a pilot study', *Nurse Education in Practice*, 31, pp. 20–28.

Feo, R., Frensham, L., Conroy, T. and Kitson, A. (2019) 'It's just common sense': Preconceptions and myths regarding fundamental care, *Nurse Education in Practice*, 36, pp. 82–84.

Fernandes, M.I., and Moreira, I.M. (2013) 'Ethical issues experienced by intensive care unit nurses in everyday practice', *Nursing Ethics*, 20(1), pp. 72–82.

Flannery, L., Ramjan, L. M., and Peters, K. (2016) 'End-of-life decisions in the Intensive Care Unit (ICU) – Exploring the experiences of ICU nurses and doctors – A critical literature review', *Australian Critical Care*, 29(2), pp. 97–103.

Gezginci, E., Goktas, S., and Orhan, B. N. (2022) 'The effects of environmental stressors in intensive care unit on anxiety and depression', *Nursing in Critical Care*, 27(1), pp. 113–119.

Greenwood, J. (1993) 'Reflective practice: a critique of the work of Argyris and Schön', *Journal of advanced nursing*, 18(8), pp. 1183–1187.

Hawkins, P. and Schwenk, G., (2011) 'The seven-eyed model of coaching supervision. Coaching and mentoring supervision', *Theory and Practice*, pp. 28–40.

Henderson, V. (1964) 'The Nature of nursing', *American Journal of Nursing*, 64, pp. 62–68.

Ingram, R., and Kautz, D.D. (2012) 'When the patient and family just do not get it: overcoming low Health Literacy in critical care', *Dimensions of Critical Care Nursing*, 31(1), pp. 25–30.

Inoue, S., Hatakeyama, J., Kondo, Y., Hifumi, T., Sakuramoto, H., Kawasaki, T., Taito, S., Nakamura, K., Unoki, T., Kawai, Y. and Kenmotsu, Y., 2019. Post-intensive care syndrome: its pathophysiology, prevention, and future directions. *Acute Medicine & Surgery*, 6(3), pp. 233–246.

International Council of Nurses (2021) 'The ICN Code of ethics for nurses'. Available at: www.icn.ch/system/files/2021-10/ICN_Code-of-Ethics_EN_Web_0.pdf (Accessed: 12 April 2023).

Jakimowicz, S., and Perry, L. (2015) 'A concept analysis of patient-centred nursing in the intensive care unit', *Journal of Advanced Nursing*, 71(7), pp. 1499–1517.

Karlsson, L., Rosenqvist, J., Airosa, F., Henricson, M., Karlsson, A.C., and Elmqvist, C. (2022) 'The meaning of caring touch for healthcare professionals in an intensive care unit: A qualitative interview study', *Intensive and Critical Care Nursing*, 68, pp. 1–7.

Kitson, A., Athlin, A. and Conroy, T. (2014) 'Anything but Basic: Nursing's challenge in meeting patients Fundamental Care Needs', *Journal of Nursing Scholarship,* 46(5), pp. 331–339.

Kitson, A., Carr, D., Conroy, T., Feo, R., Gronkjaer, M., Huisman-de Waal, G., Jackson, D., Jeffs, L., Merkley, J., Athlin, A., Parr, J., Richards, D.A., Sorensen, E.E., and Wengstorm, Y. (2019) 'Speaking up for Fundamental Care: the ILC Aalborg Statement', *BMJ Open,* 9, pp. 1–6.

Kitson, A., Conroy, T., Kuluski, K., Locock, L., and Lyons, R. (2013) 'Reclaiming and redefining the Fundamentals of Care: Nursing's response to meeting patients' basic human needs'. Available at: https://hekyll.services.adelaide.edu.au/dspace/bitstream/2440/75843/1/hdl_75843.pdf (Accessed 12 April 2023).

Kourkouta, L. (2014), 'Papathanasiou IV: Communication in nursing practice', *Mater Sociomed,* 26(1), pp. 65–67.

Lawton, S., and Shepherd, E. (2019) 'The underlying principles and procedure for bed bathing patients', *Nursing Times,* 115, pp. 5–45.

Lehman, B.J., David, D.M., and Gruber, J.A. (2017) 'Rethinking the biopsychosocial model of health: Understanding health as a dynamic system', *Social and Personality Psychology Compass, 11*(8), pp. 1–17.

Lister, L. (2022) 'Delivering compassionate care in nursing', *Practice Nursing,* 33(10), pp. 422–426.

Luce, J.M. (2010) 'End-of-life decision making in the intensive care unit', *American Journal of Respiratory and Critical Care Medicine,* 182(1), pp. 6–11.

Maslow, A.H. (1954) *Motivation and Personality.* New York: Harper and Row.

Minton, C., Batten, L., and Huntington, A. (2018) 'The impact of a prolonged stay in the ICU on patients' fundamental care needs', *Journal of Clinical Nursing,* 27(11–12), pp. 2300–2310.

Moran, F., Bradley, J.M., and Piper, A. J. (2017) 'Non-invasive ventilation for cystic fibrosis'. Available at: www.ncbi.nlm.nih.gov/pmc/articles/PMC6464053/pdf/CD002769.pdf (Accessed: 12 April 2023).

Mudd, A., Feo, R., Conroy, T., and Kitson, A. (2020) 'Where and how does fundamental car fit within seminal nursing theories: a narrative review and synthesis of key nursing concepts', *Journal of Clinical Nursing,* 29, pp. 3652–3666.

Nelson, A.M. (2014) 'Best practice in nursing: a concept analysis', *International Journal of Nursing Studies,* 51(11), pp. 1507–1516.

Romare, C., Anderberg, P., Berglund, J.S., and Skär, L. (2022) 'Burden of care related to monitoring patient vital signs during intensive care; a descriptive retrospective database study', *Intensive and Critical Care Nursing,* 71, pp. 1–7.

Roulin, M. J., and Spirig, R. (2006) 'Developing a care program to better know the chronically critically ill', *Intensive and Critical Care Nursing,* 22(6), pp. 355–361.

Ryder, M., Kitson, A., Slotnes O'Brien, T., and Timmins, F. (2021) 'Advancing nursing practice through fundamental care delivery', *Journal Nursing Management,* 30, pp. 601–603.

Schön, D (1983) *The Reflective Practitioner: How Professionals Think in Action.* New York: Basic Books.

Schön, D. (1987) *Educating the Reflective Practitioner.* San Francisco: Jossey-Bass.

Scott, J.B. (2019) Ventilators for noninvasive ventilation in adult acute care, *Respiratory Care,* 64(6), pp. 712–722.

Seaman, J. (2008) 'Experience, reflect, critique: The end of the 'learning cycles' era', *Journal of Experiential Education,* 31(1), pp. 3–18.

Stretch, B., and Shepherd, S. J. (2021) 'Criteria for intensive care unit admission and severity of illness', *Surgery,* 39(1), pp. 22–28.

Vincent, J.L., and De Backer, D. (2013) 'Circulatory shock'. *New England Journal of Medicine,* 369(18), pp. 1726–1734.

Wallbank, S. (2013) 'Maintaining professional resilience through group restorative supervision', *Community Practitioner,* 86(8), pp. 26–28.

Williams, K., Wooliams, M., and Spiro, J. (2020) *Reflective Writing,* 2nd edition. London: Bloomsbury Academic.

Yeh, J., and Ostini, R. (2020) 'The impact of health literacy environment on patient stress: a systematic review', *BMC Public Health*, 20(1), pp. 1–14.

Young, A.J., Stephens, E., and Goldsmith, J. V. (2017) 'Family caregiver communication in the ICU: Toward a relational view of health literacy', *Journal of Family Communication*, 17(2), pp. 137–152.

Youngblut, J.M. and Brooten, D (2001) 'Evidence-based nursing practice: why is it important?', *AACN Advanced Critical Care*, 12 (4), pp. 468–476.

3 Ethics and Professionalism Pillar

Ann Gallagher, Roxanne Kennedy, Matthew Jones, Helen Smith, Lisa Reynolds, and Patrick Coniam

Introduction

A commitment to understanding and enacting ethics in nursing practice is neither new nor novel (Fowler, 2016, 2021). Nurses, and other scholars, have long reflected on the many interesting and important ethical issues that inevitably arise in relationships with care-recipients, families, colleagues, communities, and organisational cultures.

Changes in our local and global communities and environment urge consideration of many new and enduring ethical challenges. Challenges relating to, for example: the climate crisis (see Chapter 6); to infectious diseases and pandemics; to demographic changes and multi-morbidities, to care workforce shortages and professional migration, to technological developments (including artificial intelligence); and to ongoing inequalities which require nurse leaders to enact a commitment to social justice.

In this chapter, we introduce ethical aspects of the anonymised scenario of Brenda McCarthy, an older person who recently moved from home to hospital to residential care. We reflect on the concept of 'home' and provide an overview of some of the most common ethical challenges that may arise in care practices. This enables readers to distinguish among ethical dilemmas, moral distress, moral injury, moral fanaticism and amoralism. Approaches to ethics provide the tools for ethical reflection which underpins nurses' accountability, and we introduce some of the most common approaches, namely: duty-based ethics (enshrined in professional codes); rights-based ethics; consequence-based ethics; virtue ethics; care ethics; and the four principles' approach. We include an overview of the meaning and implications of professionalism in contexts of complexity, ambiguity, and uncertainty.

Insights from empirical ethics, philosophical ethics, and meta-ethics, as well as from scholarship relating to professionalism – utilising the ETHICS deliberative framework – will be applied to the scenario. We also refer to codes and professional guidance from regulators in different cultural contexts and to debates relating to ethics and professionalism in contemporary nursing practice. We draw attention to scholarship and research which highlights the role of ethical/moral climate in supporting or undermining ethical nursing practice. We conclude with learning points which aim to promote learning and development in relation to ethics and professionalism.

DOI: 10.4324/9781003390565-3

Scenario: Brenda McCarthy – Ethical Decision-Making in Residential Care

Brenda McCarthy is 85 years old and a resident in a nursing home in the south of England. Nursing homes are care facilities where people live with others in later years and/or with disabilities where support is available from care-givers as needed. There are usually individual or shared bedrooms and bathrooms, as well as shared dining and activity areas.

Brenda's physical and mental health deteriorated following the death of her husband, Michael, five years ago. Brenda and Michael met and married in England in the 1960s when they worked in a local hospital where Brenda was a nurse, and Michael a porter. They both loved dancing and socialising and were well-known in the community.

Brenda's daughter, Lizzie, who lives locally, had become increasingly concerned about Brenda's safety due to her memory difficulties. Brenda would go shopping and require help from neighbours and shop owners, who had known her for many years, to find her way home. During one shopping trip, Brenda had a fall and was admitted to hospital with a fracture.

As Brenda was recovering in hospital, Lizzie and brother, Stephen, had an online meeting to discuss Brenda's future care. Lizzie was of the view that Brenda was unsafe at home and said she was unable to give Brenda the care she needed. Lizzie had a part-time job and was caring for two grandchildren three days a week. Lizzie's daughter, Maggie, experiences depression and at times becomes overwhelmed, needing the support of her mother to assist with childcare. Stephen lives locally, has poor health and admits he wants 'a quiet life' and 'no hassle'. He leaves decision-making, regarding his mother's care, to his sister. The hospital team made it clear that they wanted to discharge Brenda as they did not have sufficient beds for patients admitted. Lizzie approached her mother about a move to a care home and, following a visit to the local care home, Brenda reluctantly agreed to a transfer for a trial period.

Admission to the care home was stressful for Brenda as she was sad to leave her home of 65 years. However, she settled well initially and made friends with some of the other residents. Brenda particularly enjoyed activities such as bingo and singing. The multi-cultural care home team includes care-givers from the Philippines, India and Nigeria. Brenda is particularly fond of Amma in particular, a care-giver from Ghana. Brenda's daughter, Lizzie, visits frequently.

Recently, Brenda seems increasingly confused. A holistic assessment confirms that she is experiencing dementia. She repeatedly says 'I want to go home'. Amma observes that staff respond to Brenda's question inconsistently, with some telling Brenda that there is no transport today as it is Sunday (even when it is not). Amma does not think these responses are ethical or professional and feels very uncomfortable about a lack of honesty in the team regarding communication with residents. She is also increasingly concerned about staff shortages and often leaves work feeling that she is not providing the care she would like to, believing she is 'cutting corners' and neglecting some residents. Amma is aware that home manager and registered nurse, Gordon, is an enthusiast for technology and overheard a conversation between Gordon, talking with a technology company representative, about the introduction of 'carebots' into the care home.

Ethics in Nursing Practice

Nursing is a moral and relational practice which goes beyond clinical aspects of well-being and recovery. Nursing requires the enactment of moral attitudes that underpin the way nurses undertake and perform tasks. Care activities, such as assistance with personal hygiene or administering medication, cannot be reduced to technical or physical behaviours. Instead, they are enveloped in the caring and trusting relationships built between nurse and care-recipient, relationships which are necessary to support patient's dignity (Gastmans, 1999).

Ethics – also known as moral philosophy – is not a recently invented discipline but has been pondered over for thousands of years. The word 'ethics' was derived from the Greek phrase 'ethos', meaning character and the 'science of morals'. The word 'morality' has origins in Old French and Latin with meanings ranging from moral instruction, character to goodness or virtuousness (Online Etymology Dictionary, no date). Some argue that there is a distinct difference between morality and ethics, with morality relating to personal values and ethics representing a formal discipline and universal codes with requirements such as 'do no harm' (Harper, 2009). Others suggest that the philosophical distinction is simply down to language, and to separate the two generates further ambiguity as they both relate to right and wrong behaviour (Johnstone, 2019). For the purposes of this chapter, we take the view that morality refers to the values, beliefs and opinions that anyone can hold or demonstrate, without the need to understand underpinning theory or evolution of the field. 'Ethics', on the other hand, refers to an academic discipline, providing philosophical and empirical perspectives on 'morality'.

There is a substantial literature on nursing ethics dating back to the 19th century. Professor Marsha Fowler (2016) reports that, over 400 articles on the theme of nursing ethics were published between 1900 and 1965 in the *American Journal of Nursing*. There were also 50 books on nursing ethics, authored by nurses, philosophers and theologians, published between the 1890s and the 1960s. Professor Fowler (2016, p. 7) argues:

> The key to understanding the moral identity of modern nursing and the distinctiveness of nursing ethics resides in a deeper examination of the extensive nursing ethics literature and history from the late 1800s to the mid 1960s, prior to the 'bioethics revolution'. There is a distinctive nursing ethics, but one that falls outside both biomedical and bioethics and is larger than either.

Debate continues as to whether nursing ethics is a distinctive field and how it relates to bioethics, medical ethics and other examples of applied and professional ethics. Does, for example, nursing ethics warrant different theoretical or normative approaches to ethics? Whereas early professional ethics prioritised good moral character and virtues such as loyalty and obedience, contemporary ethics is much more diverse with many different philosophical underpinnings. Overall, nursing ethics is a practice-based field that describes and prescribes the value base of nursing. It involves the processes of learning, examining and preserving values and principles, underpinned by what is right and wrong and maintaining high-quality patient care (Haddad and Geiger, 2022).

Ethics is the universal term used when examining and understanding how to behave and live within a moral code of what is considered acceptable or unacceptable (Johnstone, 2019). Understanding the different types or categories of ethics enables us to appreciate the ways nursing ethics contributes to everyday nursing, enabling reflection on care-giving practice. There are three main types or categories of ethics: empirical or descriptive ethics; philosophical or prescriptive ethics; and metaethics.

Empirical or descriptive ethics involves describing the moral life through qualitative and quantitative research such as, for example, nurses' experiences of ethical dilemmas, care-recipients' perspectives on dignity in care, nurse managers' views of organisational ethical culture and measurements of phenomena such as moral distress and moral courage.

Philosophical or prescriptive ethics involves consideration and application of principles and theories that guide nursing practice. They equip us with the tools to reflect on our practice and to uphold accountability in providing arguments for our actions and omissions.

Metaethics is concerned with the meaning of ethical concepts such as 'autonomy', 'responsibility', 'compassion' or 'privacy' and enables us to better understand ethical conflicts that nurses may experience in practice.

What Ethics Is and What It Is Not

There is sometimes confusion as to how ethics relates to other frameworks that impact decision-making and behaviour, for example, law and religion. Ethics is not the same as law, and although there is overlap, the differences need to be understood. Historical examples which conflict with ethical principles include laws imposed during apartheid, which enforced racial discrimination in South Africa (Revell, 2017; Coldwell, 2017) and laws during the Nazi era which contributed to unethical biomedical experimentation and genocide (Steinweis and Rachlin, 2013). There remain contemporary laws which contribute to inequality relating to race, class, gender and age and which result in harm, discrimination, indignity and disrespect. Ethics enables us to critique, and take a stand against, laws which violate human rights, preferences, well-being and interests.

Ethics is also not the same as religion. Nurses, and other health and care professions, embrace many different faith perspectives or none at all (Gallagher and Herbert, 2019). While many religious and humanistic values and/or beliefs are compatible with nursing ethics, some may lead to nurses experiencing ethical conflict (see Chapter 7).

The next section explores some of the most common Western perspectives on nursing ethics. We wish to emphasise that perspectives from, for example, Indigenous communities, from the East and from the Global South, are not represented in the approaches outlined below. It is important that nurses engage with approaches to ethics which are best suited to their professional and cultural context and not accept, uncritically, perspectives which are less well suited. That said, ethical frameworks such as human rights are applicable across cultures and the International Council of Nurses Code (International Council of Nurses, 2021) provides guidance to nurses everywhere.

Approaches to Ethics

Scholarship in philosophical ethics provides nurses and other care-givers with frameworks which help to better understand, and respond to, ethical aspects of practice. Approaches to ethics enable nurses to consider different lenses to analyse practice situations. While there are many potential approaches to philosophical nursing ethics, we will consider six of the most common approaches and a more recent approach which brings together key elements of ethics in relation to the art of care:

- *Rights-based ethics* – increasing attention has been paid to rights in health and social care practices, particularly in relation to people in minority and marginalised groups. For example, people who are older, refugees or who experience mental distress or learning disabilities. For rights to be meaningful, it is necessary for there to be duties – on the part of individuals, groups or governments – to respect these rights. In relation to the scenario above, we need to consider the rights of each person involved. There has, for example, been recent attention to the rights of older people in relation to the COVID-19 pandemic (Amnesty International, 2020).
- *Duty-based ethics* – also referred to as deontology (from *deon* [duty] and *logos* [study of]) – which focuses on nurses' duties or obligations (Rawling, 2023) towards care-recipients, families and communities. Codes of conduct or relating to ethics are often framed in terms of duties with, for example, statements which begin with 'should', 'ought' or 'must'. In the discussion of 'professionalism' below, we discuss the role of professional codes which guide the practice of registered nurses such as Gordon in the scenario.
- *Consequence-based ethics* – an example of which is utilitarianism (Mill, 1863; Sevier, 2021) – focuses on weighing benefits and harms with a view to bringing about the 'most good' or most benefit for the most people or 'the greatest happiness of the greatest number' (Crimmins, 2021). Nurses in public health who manage budgets or scarce resources during a pandemic, for example, will be acutely aware of decision-making at the level of groups or populations rather than focusing on the needs of individual care-recipients (Savulescu et al., 2020). Introducing technology into Brenda's care home may lead registered nurse, Gordon, to weigh the benefits and harms or risks of introducing technologies such as carebots (Gallagher et al., 2016).
- *Virtue ethics* – whereas the approaches above focus on the conduct and decision-making of nurses and other care-givers, a virtue ethics approach focuses on their character. Qualities of character, or virtues, required for nursing practice include care, courage, respectfulness, integrity, justice and professional wisdom (Banks and Gallagher, 2009). In the scenario above, Amma's concerns suggest that she enacts virtues of care, respectfulness, and honesty as she reflects on Brenda's care, particularly in relation to truth-telling.
- *Care ethics* – a more recent approach, which dates back to the scholarship of Carol Gilligan (1982) and Nel Noddings (1984), has assumed a central role in nursing ethics (Gallagher, 2017). This approach focuses on the relationships developed between care-givers and care-recipients and on concepts such as dependence, dignity and non-abandonment which are relevant to care-givers responses to Brenda above.
- *The four principles approach* – debate continues as to which is the most helpful and appropriate approach to nursing ethics. Some nurse ethicists, for example, Fowler (2021) consider the biomedical origins of the four principles' approach to be unsuitable

for nursing ethics. However, the four principles' approach is one of the most common approaches and is, arguably, a useful way to frame and underpin nursing decisions. The four principles are: respect for autonomy; non-maleficence (do not harm); beneficence (do good); and justice (treat people fairly). All four principles require reflection on the implications of each principle and a balancing which is described as 'reflective equilibrium' (Gillon, 1986; Beauchamp and Childress, 2019; Edwards, 2009).

A more recent approach to facilitate reflection on ethical aspects of care practices is *slow ethics* (Gallagher, 2020). This approach builds on insights from the 'slow movement' (Honoré, 2005) and encourages reflection on: sensitivity; solidarity; scholarship; sustainability; space; and stories.

Ethical Challenges in Care Practices

Ethics is integral to nurses' relationships with care-recipients, families, communities, colleagues and managers. Nurses are entrusted to deliver care to people when at their most vulnerable. They work to prevent ill-health, to enable recovery and, when the latter is not possible, nurses prioritise the best possible end of life experience. Much nursing practice is ethically unproblematic with nurses acting ethically and demonstrating good character. For example, nurses provide information so people can make informed choices. They maintain confidentiality and prioritise respect for human dignity and demonstrate a wide range of ethical qualities or virtues and adherence to principles, rights and duties as outlined above.

A wide range of ethical challenges also arise in everyday nursing practice. Challenges that relate to nurses' engagement with individuals, organisations, systems and the environment. Nurses may feel challenged, for example, by individual requests for, or refusal of, treatment or care (Gallagher, 2020). Individuals do not always want what nurses consider they need, nor do they always need what they request. Organisations also present ethical challenges, for example, when there are insufficient care-givers and/or when material resources to deliver good care are inadequate or when the culture or climate is unethical (see, discussion of ethical climate below).

In everyday practice, nurses experience *ethical dilemmas* when there are two equally desirable or undesirable courses of action involving a conflict of values. An example might include a situation where a person refuses care that nurses consider they need. On the one hand, nurses are committed to doing good (beneficence) and also respecting autonomy (an individual's right to make decisions about their own care and treatment including refusal) (Gallagher, 2020). Such dilemmas can also contribute to moral distress.

Research and scholarship regarding *moral distress* (McCarthy and Gastmans, 2015) has escalated in recent years due, primarily, to the ethical challenges presented by the COVID-19 pandemic. As with many concepts in nursing ethics, moral distress is contested with different definitions and different perspectives regarding helpfulness. Johnstone and Hutchinson (2015) argue that moral distress should be abandoned as it fosters victimhood. In general terms, moral distress is understood to refer to the experience of care-givers when they believe they know the right thing to do but are unable to do it. Health and social care systems which do not have, for example, sufficient staff or beds compromise good care and can result in nurses experiencing moral distress. This appears to be the experience of Amma in the scenario. Enduring moral distress can result in burnout and nurses leaving the profession.

Other moral challenges which nurses might experience or observe in others can include: *moral injury* when individuals' integrity is undermined by experiences of unethical practice resulting in guilt or shame (Čartolovni et al., 2021). Nurses may also experience *ethical unpreparedness* when they feel ill-equipped to think through and respond to ethical issues in practice. More unusual ethical challenges that nurses may encounter are *amoralism*, whereby individuals lack commitment to ethics in practice, and *moral fanaticism* when individuals focus on one outcome (Johnstone, 2019). An example of moral fanaticism is where a practitioner is intent on resuscitation, regardless of whether it is in accord with the care-recipients' wishes or is futile.

Awareness of the range of ethical challenges that may be encountered in health and social care practices enables nurses and other care-givers to understand better what ethical practice means. This understanding contributes to an appreciation of what it means to be a professional in contexts of complexity, uncertainty and ambiguity as in the scenario of Brenda above, to which we turn next.

Professionalism: What Does it Mean? And Why Does it Matter?

The etymology of the word 'profession' suggests it has multiple origins, part Latin and part French. In early uses, 'profession' was synonymous with the professions of law, the church, and medicine. Its earliest uses relate to the declaration of faith and principles, and to vows taken when entering a religious order (Oxford English Dictionary, 2022).

There is no clear consensus on what professionalism means in care practices, however, it is likely that readers will have ideas and opinions about what it means and what actions denote professional or unprofessional behaviours. Some widely agreed attributes of professionalism include: appearance and behaviour, underpinning knowledge and experience, accountability, abiding by an institutional framework of professional conduct and adherence to ethical and moral codes, alongside providing a service with respect and dignity to the beneficiary (Wagner et al., 2007).

In addition to reflecting on the meaning and implications of professionalism in nursing practice, it is important to define the purpose of professionalism. For example, what and who is *professionalism* for? In health care, the beneficiaries of the service are patients, however, patients' perspectives are often lost in the narrative regarding what it means to be a professional (Bulk et al., 2019). Patients' perspectives vary on what they consider the most important aspects of professionalism, and these are largely dependent on the type of healthcare setting (Lynch et al., 2004).

Many factors influence nurses' perceptions of, and aspirations to, professionalism in their everyday practice including personal experience of giving and receiving care, role models in care contexts; and their educational preparation. Kelly (2020), for example, discusses the impact of 'the hidden curriculum', whereby undergraduate nursing students' are influenced by factors outside the formal curriculum such as core values developed at a young age, the witnessing of role model behaviour and the formation of core values and ethical principles based on cultural and social norms. In addition to reflecting on professionalism and ethics in nursing practice, nurses need also to be informed by evidence, this is an integral part of professionalism in care settings (see Chapter 4). In addition to engaging with scholarship relating to ethics and professionalism, guidance on professional conduct and character is also detailed in codes of conduct and ethics. We turn to these next.

Ethics, Professionalism, and the Role of Codes

The first international Code of Ethics for nurses was published by the International Council of Nurses (ICN) in 1953. The Preamble to the current ICN Code states:

> From the origins of organised nursing in the mid-1800s and recognising nursing care is deeply rooted in the traditions and practices of equity and inclusion and the appreciation of diversity, nurses have consistently recognised four fundamental nursing responsibilities: to promote health, to prevent illness, to restore health, and to alleviate suffering and promote a dignified death. The need for nursing is universal.
>
> (International Council of Nurses, 2021, p. 2)

The current Code reminds of its purpose:

> The ICN Code of Ethics for Nurses is a statement of the ethical values, responsibilities and professional accountabilities of nurses and nursing students that defines and guides ethical nursing practice within the different roles nurses assume. It is not a code of conduct but can serve as a framework for ethical nursing practice and decision-making to meet professional standards set by regulatory bodies.
>
> (International Council of Nurses, 2021, p. 2)

The Code is described as 'a guide for action based on social values and needs. It will have meaning only as a living document if applied to the realities of nursing and health care in all settings in which nursing is delivered' (International Council of Nurses, 2021, p. 4). It has 4 elements, which make explicit priorities regarding nurses' wide-ranging ethical obligations in relation to: 'nurses and patients or other people requiring care or services, nurses and practice, nurses and the profession, and nurses and global health' (International Council of Nurses, 2021, p. 3).

In addition to guidance from the ICN Code of Ethics nurses and students of nursing, in many countries, need also to reflect on, and act in accord with, country-specific codes. The UK Nursing and Midwifery Council (NMC) Code, for example, has four key elements: prioritise people; practise effectively; preserve safety; and promote professionalism and trust (Nursing and Midwifery Council, 2018). Each section of the NMC Code needs to be reflected on – and enacted – by nurses and nursing students, in relation to their care practices.

The final section of the NMC Code 'promote professionalism and trust' outlines a registered nurse's responsibility to be 'a model of integrity and leadership' which will in turn, gain the trust of patients and colleagues. In addition to this, in 2017, the four chief nursing officers of the UK, with support from the NMC launched a comprehensive guide on professionalism for nurses which elaborates the NMC's professional standards and expectations of registered nurses. The authors of 'Enabling Professionalism' state:

> It is recognised that nurses and midwives work in a range of environments in organisations. It is the organisations that, in many cases, are responsible for systems and processes that enable professional practice, rather than individual practice areas.
>
> (Nursing and Midwifery Council, 2017, p. 6).

Whereas much historical scholarship on nursing ethics focused on the conduct and character of individual nurses, more recent discussions have highlighted the importance of organisational culture in supporting or undermining nurses' ethical practice.

Ethics and Organisational Culture

There have been too many historical and contemporary reports of unethical care practices internationally. While some of these can be attributed solely to the actions and omissions of individual practitioners, organisational culture makes a significant contribution. One of the most significant and tragic care failures in the United Kingdom, in recent times, relates to the Mid Staffordshire NHS Foundation Trust. Robert Francis QC who led the investigation wrote, in the executive summary (Francis, 2013, p. 3) to one of the reports:

> the story it tells is one of appalling suffering of many patients. This was primarily caused by a serious failure on the part of a provider Trust Board. It did not listen sufficiently to its patients and staff or ensure the correction of deficiencies brought to the Trust's attention. Above all, it failed to tackle an insidious negative culture involving a tolerance of poor standards and a disengagement from managerial and leadership responsibilities. This failure was in part the consequence of allowing a focus on reaching national access targets, achieving financial balance and seeking foundation trust status to be at the cost of delivering acceptable standards of care.

Much attention is now paid to the contribution organisations play in supporting or undermining ethical care practices. This is often framed as 'organisational culture' which refers to 'the collective beliefs, assumptions, ideas, and approaches developed by a group of professionals that informs how they interact with each other and the methods they apply to overcome obstacles' (Glassdoor, 2021). Ethical climate or moral climate focuses on a type of organisational culture, where there are shared perceptions of ethical behaviour and how ethical issues in the organisation should be responded to (Koskenvuori et al., 2018). Research in nursing ethics has demonstrated that when the ethical climate of a care organisation is good, there is likely to be less moral distress (Pauly et al., 2009). That is, when nurses are working in an organisation with a positive ethical climate, they are more likely to be able to do the right thing and to deliver good care. In terms of relevancy to Brenda, we return to the scenario below and the ethical issues which arise, most particularly, in residential care relationships.

Application of the ETHICS Framework to the Scenario

A framework which enables nurses and other care-givers to reflect on – and apply – approaches to nursing ethics is the **ETHICS** deliberative framework (Gallagher, 2008) as below:

- Enquire about the facts of the situation/case.
- Think/Talk through the options available to those involved.
- Hear the views of key stakeholders.
- Identify relevant principles and other values.
- Clarify the meaning and implications of key values.
- Select a course of action and present ethical arguments to support action.

Ethical and professional issues which arise in the scenario of Brenda, outlined at the beginning of the chapter include: family roles and responsibilities regarding care provision for older people; the introduction of technology into residential care (e.g. carebots); responses to care-givers' moral distress when resources are inadequate to deliver good care; and responses to Brenda's requests to go home. All of these areas are worthy of in-depth ethical analysis, however due to space constraints, it is possible to focus only on one ethical aspect of Brenda's care. We opted to analyse staff responses to Brenda's repeated requests to go home.

Enquire about the Facts of the Situation/Case: Who? What? How? Where? When? Why?

The scenario states that 'staff find the situation challenging as Brenda is increasingly confused and repeatedly says "I want to go home"'. Amma observes that staff members respond inconsistently, with some telling Brenda that there is no transport today as it is Sunday (even when it is not). Amma does not think these responses are ethical or professional. How should care-givers respond to Brenda's desire to go 'home'? This begs questions regarding truth-telling in response to people who appear 'confused' and who may experience dementia. Before discussing ethical aspects of truth-telling – and lying – in care, we engage with literature which explores this particular situation and possible explanation for Brenda's repeated requests to go 'home'. Interesting interpretations of the meaning of home to people experiencing dementia, drawn from qualitative research, refers to people's feelings of 'uncanniness' or 'unfamiliarity':

> where both the body and the brain are affected by the disease. The ability to orient oneself in one's surroundings is severely affected so [a person experiencing dementia] will struggle to find their way round in a world that seems more and more foreign. Moving into an institution poses an additional threat to the feeling of home because it takes the person away from their embodied and familiar environment. Research has emphasised how institutionalisation often leads to additional disorientation, which again leads to homesickness (Zingmark et al., 1993), with the institution coming across simultaneously as both hospital and home and as neither hospital nor home.
>
> (Haugen, 2020, p. 67)

Haugen (2020, p. 67) goes on to summarise research where nursing homes are described as 'refugee camps' or as 'prisons without bars' as places 'that we are unable to attach value to or that we attach a negative value to are often referred to as non-places'. Time is identified as central to people's experiences of dementia as short-term memory is impacted, leading to difficulties adjusting to people's current situation:

> Home is often placed in childhood, and many people with dementia do not seem to remember that they have grown old, and they believe that their children are still small and that their own parents are still alive. Seeing their own image in the mirror can be disturbing from some, and some end up believing that the old person in the mirror is their parent.
>
> (Haugen, 2020, p. 73)

The idea, then, of wanting to go home needs to be reflected on deeply with a wide range of interpretations. Haugen's (2020) work reminds that 'home' is 'a relational thing', a place where people leave familiar objects, as somewhere they feel at peace and alone, or perhaps as a final resting place. In relation to the people experiencing dementia, seeking 'home' has been described as attempts to find 'a solution to . . . dislocation and feelings of homesickness' (Haugen, 2020, p. 81). Haugen (2020) reminds that the suffering and distress experienced by people seeking home need to be understood and their home seeking behaviours as 'activities that matter and accomplish something' (Haugen, 2020, p. 81).

With this background, detailing the significance of 'home', of 'homesickness' and home seeking as meaningful, we move back to the Amma's concern regarding care-givers' responses to Brenda's requests to go home. This brings us to the next section of the ETHICS framework.

Think/Talk through the Options Available to Those Involved

Are the options, in response to Brenda's repeated requests to go home, only to tell the truth or to tell lies? Arguments for and against truth-telling in care are well rehearsed (see, for example, Tuckett, 2004). Scholarship by Kamphof and Hendriks (2020, p. 272) emphasises that helping people with dementia experience 'temporal "episodes of home-coming" is increasingly seen as a core task for person-centred care' and that feeling at home is something 'one *becomes*' and may also 'lose again'. This understanding forms the backdrop to reflection on responses to Brenda's repeated requests to go home. In addition to options relating to truth-telling and lying, there is need to consider truthfulness in the care home environment more broadly. What strategies to promote a homely or homelike environment are ethical? And which are not? Is, for example, the use of fake doors simulating a previous home or of dolls to simulate babies, ethically acceptable? (Kamphof and Hendriks, 2020). While care-giver verbal responses to Brenda's requests to go home are important, this needs to be considered in the context of the care home culture.

Hear the Views of Key Stakeholders (Care-Recipients, Families, Other Care-givers)

In the Scenario above, Amma was uncomfortable with the responses of other care-givers who lied to Brenda. It would be interesting to have the perspectives of Brenda, her daughter and care-givers in response to the question: should care-givers always tell the truth? Are there situations when with-holding the truth is ethically defensible? Are there alternatives to truth-telling and lying? Some caregivers, for example, argue that distraction is a more positive strategy. They might, for example, invite Brenda to participate in some meaningful activity or initiate a conversation regarding Brenda's earlier life, work as a nurse, or how she met her husband.

Identify Relevant Principles and Other Values

It has been argued that deception, which includes lying, is ethically problematic as it 'compromises the dignity and trust of people with dementia and the authenticity of life on the ward' (Kamphof and Hendriks, 2020, p. 287). Here, then, are introduced important values of dignity, trust and authenticity. The approaches to ethics outlined above present a wider range of options regarding care-giver responses to Brenda when she is requesting to go home.

An ethical analysis involving the four principles approach enables us to consider what follows from each principle in relation to Brenda's situation: respect for autonomy; beneficence; non-maleficence; and justice.

It can be argued that the most relevant virtues or moral qualities that care-givers need to demonstrate, in response to Brenda's experiences, include respectfulness, care and professional wisdom (Banks and Gallagher, 2009). Other ethical frameworks that throw light on the scenario include Codes, rights frameworks (rights to know and not to know) and care ethics. Insights from slow ethics also have relevance, focusing on the value of stories, ethical sensitivity, solidarity, scholarship, space and sustainability.

Clarify the Meaning and Implications of Key Values

An overview of the four principles approach is outlined above. However, there is more to say regarding each of these:

- **Respect for autonomy** – the concept 'autonomy' comes from Greek words *autos* (self) and *nomos* (government or rule). It is important to remember that none of us are fully autonomous, that is, there are external and internal constraints and enablers which impact our autonomy. Brenda's experience of dementia is likely to be an internal constraint and Amma's autonomy is likely to be constrained by external constraints such as resources and time. Autonomy enables us to invite and process information and to make informed decisions. The principle of autonomy is particularly important in health and social care as it underpins ethical rules such as informed consent, confidentiality and truth-telling. However, autonomy has evolved to take into account that fact that humans are in relationship with others – hence relational autonomy. The principle of respect for autonomy is considered more in keeping with cultures where individualism rather than collective approaches are paramount. Respect for autonomy relates to Brenda's ability to make decisions and to professional decision-making which enables or thwarts her decision to go home. This may also connect with legal guidance regarding capacity, for example, in accord with the United Kingdom Mental Capacity Act 2005 (Office of the Public Guardian, 2014). Readers, please check relevant law relating to capacity, in your own jurisdiction.
- **Beneficence** – the imperative to bring benefit and to 'do good' should underpin all health and social care practice in promoting the flourishing of individuals, families and communities where this is possible. In relation to Brenda's desire to go home, the benefits of truth-telling – in response to her requests to go home – versus other strategies to support her well-being need to be balanced with risks and potential harms. This principle is generally balanced with the principle of non-maleficence.
- **Non-maleficence** – this principle has a long history and is often considered the first and most important, with the dictum *primum non nocere* – above all (or, first), do no harm. Types and implication of harm' requires reflection in care practices. Harm can be, for example, physical, psychological or emotional and may be the consequence of a wide range of activities ranging, for example, from abuse, exploitation and neglect to verbal slights and being ignored or disrespected. Minimising harm to Brenda requires ethical sensitivity and person-centredness, alongside weighing benefits of different responses to her requests to go home.
- **Justice** – this is a complex and wide-ranging principle which includes the fair distribution of resources (for example, care-giver time); non-discriminatory practices (not

treating people of different ages, cultures, gender or with other protected features, unfairly). In relation to Brenda, we need to be particularly mindful of discrimination on grounds of age or disability.

In addition to the four principles, summarised above, it is important to consider also the most relevant virtues or moral qualities that care-givers need to demonstrate, in response to Brenda's experiences. Minimally, these include respectfulness, care and professional wisdom. Other ethical frameworks that throw light on the scenario include professional codes, rights frameworks (rights to know and not to know) and care ethics.

Select a Course of Action and Present Ethical Arguments to Support Action

Chapter authors – four with experience as family carers of people experiencing dementia – discussed the most ethical response to Brenda's requests to go home. One author reflected on her own challenging experience of caring for a parent who had dementia and intention to do good and alleviate the distress of a loved one:

> Looking back, I wished we had been more honest in some respects and also, told more lies. I think we should have been more honest with telling her about the dementia, but once it had got to a point were understanding of where home was or where people were, it was in the best interest to lie. Mum wanted to go home, but really, she wanted to go back to being safe, and a well time, and home from her changed as the dementia got worse. The fear she had, scared that her mum and dad were ill and in hospital and she wanted to get word to them, we decided to lie and say that we had been in contact with them. This gave her peace and reassurance, no benefit to her to say they both died over 40 years ago.

Family members make decisions which may run counter to their usual ethical intuitions. The experience of dementia and the distress that may impact the older person may lead to conclusions, as above, that harm and distress should be minimised (non-maleficence). They may engage in what is called 'therapeutic lying', that is, lying intended to benefit the person. In the professional sphere, it has been argued that this should be a 'last resort' (Learner, 2015).

Engagement with Brenda's emotions, and distraction with meaningful activity including conversation and hobbies, were considered the most ethically defensible approaches. Lying and deception were not, generally, considered ethical nor in keeping with the ethos or moral climate of a care facility that focuses on ethical practice and professionalism. It is important that care planning is a collaborative process with ethical responses agreed.

Ethical Competence?

An important question which relates to education in relation to each of the 7 Pillars discussed in this book is: what will success look like? That is, what are we aiming towards as we promote learning in relation to each Pillar? The Pillar 'Ethics and Professionalism' suggests that success relates to people doing the right thing and being good nurses, however, we agreed that this is a broad and deep endeavour involving the demonstration of ethical competence in care practices.

The moral life is complex, and it is helpful to break down the elements of ethical – or moral – competence. An integrative review concluded that while there is no consensus, there are common elements of ethical competence (Lechasseur et al., 2018). An example of a model for reflection on elements of ethical competence was suggested by one of the authors (Gallagher, 2006). The elements of this model include: ethical seeing/perception; ethical knowing; ethical reflection; ethical doing; and ethical being.

Ethical Seeing/Perception

One of the ethical challenges encountered in care practices is that of moral blindness, whereby people are aware of clinical or technical aspects of care, and insensitive to ethical aspects such as the principles and virtues discussed above. Ethical 'seeing' requires finely honed skills in listening and perceiving people's needs and desires. For example, in relation to the Scenario, it is critical to reflect on the meaning of 'home' for Brenda and to notice the impact of more and less respectful responses, as Amma demonstrated.

Immersive simulation and workshops which enable students to observe, listen carefully may assist with the development of skills in ethical perception (Gallagher et al., 2017, 2020).

Ethical Knowing

When reflecting on ethics and professionalism in care practices, it is necessary to have knowledge of different approaches and to be able to integrate – or apply – ethical frameworks to care situations.

Having a good working knowledge of approaches to ethics such as: principles, virtues, rights, duties and consequentialist approaches, enable nurses to demonstrate accountability in justifying actions and omissions. Engaging with peers and educators in online and face to face education are strategies also to enhance ethical knowing.

Ethical Reflection

Throughout this text, readers are introduced to a number of reflective frameworks. In this chapter, we introduced the ETHICS deliberative framework. Reflecting 'in action' and on 'action' are equally important in relation to ethical competence.

Ethical Doing

Doing the right thing by care-recipients, families, and communities is necessarily a core focus in nursing ethics. Nurses' actions and omissions impact other people in both positive and negative ways. Role modelling and inviting feedback are important strategies in promoting and sustaining ethical conduct (Hunter and Cook, 2018).

Ethical Being

The aspiration to *be* good or virtuous is a central feature of virtue ethics, underpinned by the awareness that we are flawed and fallible humans. We can take stock of virtues we demonstrate and how we continue to refine and develop our practice as 'good nurses'. We need also to consider how we develop the resilience needed to sustain and develop ethical nursing and leadership practices (Monteverde, 2014).

Conclusion

This chapter introduces the Ethics and Professionalism Pillar of Learning, focusing on the experience of an older person, Brenda McCarthy, and her care-givers. We provided an overview of ethical challenges that may arise in care practices which included: ethical dilemmas, moral distress, moral blindness, moral injury, moral fanaticism and amoralism. We provide a summary of different approaches to ethics which included duty-based ethics; rights-based ethics; consequence-based ethics; virtue ethics; care ethics; and the four principles' approach. We referred to codes and professional guidance from regulators and advise engagement with local Codes in different cultural contexts. We highlight the role of ethical/moral climate in supporting or undermining ethical nursing practice.

We hope that this overview of the Ethics and Professional Pillar of Learning will enable readers to reflect on and develop ethical competence in nursing practice, leadership and research. Ethics is too often considered an esoteric and lofty discipline removed from the everyday. We hope we have demonstrated in this chapter that ethics is integral to who we are and what we do in professional and personal life. It is our view that if we engage with and apply ethics appropriately in our care practices, excellent care will follow with: care-recipients, families, and communities being enabled to flourish; care-givers being valued and nurse leaders role modelling exemplary ethical behaviour, showing the way to care practices we will be proud of and wish to celebrate.

Takeaways for Student Nurses

- Ethics is concerned with doing the right thing, with being of good character and with the development and sustainability of positive relationships with other humans, other species and the environment.
- Nursing is a moral and relational practice concerned with promoting the flourishing of individuals, families and communities and an aspiration to excellence in health and social care.
- A wide range of approaches to ethics assist with deliberation and decision-making in nursing practice, leadership and research. These include: rights-based ethics; duty-based ethics; consequence-based ethics; virtue ethics; and the four principles approach. These need to be contextualised within specific cultural and professional contexts with reflection on appropriateness and applicability to practice situations.
- Ethical competence includes elements such as: ethical seeing or perception; ethical knowing, ethical reflection, ethical doing or conduct and ethical being or character. These elements require ongoing self-evaluation with support from peers, educators and members of multi-professional teams in health and social care practice.
- Student nurses should prioritise availing of opportunities to engage meaningfully with individuals, families, communities and cultures to better understand – and value – different needs, desires and perspectives.

- Student nurses are well placed to create opportunities to engage in discussion regarding past, current and future ethical issues which impact health and social care practice. They should demonstrate a commitment to listening to and learning from diverse perspectives and demonstrate curiosity, humility and open-mindedness as you strive to be the best you can be as future nurse leaders.

Takeaways for educators/practitioners

- Value the significant impact of your experience and expertise as a nurse educator, practitioner and researcher to positively influence nurse leaders of the future.
- Reflect on the ways your role modelling in everyday nursing practice, leadership, education and research influences the actions and omissions of student nurses, peers and other professions.
- Make time and reflective spaces to stimulate student nurses' curiosity and open-mindedness and to explore ethical aspects of nursing practice, creating opportunities for students to better appreciate complexity and the importance of person- and family-centredness.
- Explore with students how elements of ethical competence manifest in everyday nursing practice, leadership, education and research and how they can develop and sustain ethical practice.
- Take time to reflect on and develop moral resilience which enables you to be restored and better appreciate your important contribution to the flourishing of students, care-recipients, families and organisational culture.

References

Amnesty International (2020) *As if Expendable: The UK Government's Failure to Protect Older People in Care Homes during the COVID-19 Pandemic*. London: Amnesty International.

Banks, S. and Gallagher, A. (2009) *Ethics in Professional Life: Virtues for Health and Social Care*. Basingstoke: Palgrave Macmillan.

Beauchamp, T.L. and Childress, J.F. (2019) *Principles of Biomedical Ethics*, 8th edn. New York: Oxford University Press.

Bulk, L.Y., Drynan, D., Murphy, S., Gerber, P., Bezati, R., Trivett, S. and Jarus, T. (2019) 'Patient perspectives: four pillars of professionalism', *Patient Experience Journal*, 6(3), pp. 74–81.

Čartolovni, A., Stolt, M. and Rancare Cost Action. (2021) 'Moral injury in healthcare professionals: A scoping review and discussion', *Nursing Ethics*, 28(5), pp. 590–602. Available at: https://doi.org/10.1177/0969733020966

Coldwell, D. (2017) 'Apartheid and Ethics', in D. Poff and A. Michalos (eds) *Encyclopedia of Business and Professional Ethics*. s.l., Springer Cham, pp. 1–5.

Crimmins, J.E. (2021) Jeremy Bentham, *Stanford Encyclopaedia of Philosophy*, 1 December. Available at: https://plato.stanford.edu/entries/bentham/ (Accessed 2 April 2023).

Edwards, S.D. (2009) *Nursing Ethics: A Principle-Based Approach*. 2nd edn. Basingstoke: Palgrave MacMillan.

Fowler M.D. (2016) 'Heritage ethics: Toward a thicker account of nursing ethics', *Nursing Ethics*, 23(1), pp. 7–21.

Fowler, M.D. (2021) 'Toward reclaiming our ethical heritage: Nursing ethics before bioethics', *The Online Journal of Issues in Nursing (OJIN)*, 25(04). Available at: https://ojin.nursingworld.org/MainMenuCategories/ANAMarketplace/ANAPeriodicals/OJIN/TableofContents/Vol-25-2020/No2-May-2020/Toward-Reclaiming-Our-Ethical-Heritage-Nursing-Ethics-before-Bioethics.html (Accessed 4 April 2023).

Francis, R. (2013) *Report of the Mid Staffordshire NHS Foundation Trust Public Inquiry: Executive summary* [online]. Norwich: The Stationary Office. Available at: https://assets.publishing.service.gov.uk/government/uploads/system/uploads/attachment_data/file/279124/0947.pdf (Accessed 2 March 2023).

Gallagher, A. (2006) 'Promoting Ethical Competence'. In A.J. Davis, V. Tschudin and De Raeve (eds), *The Teaching of Nursing Ethics: Content and Methods*. Edinburgh: Elsevier, pp. 223–239.

Gallagher, A. (2008) 'Block 3: Introducing ethics in health and social care'. In *A181 Ethics in Real Life*. Milton Keynes, The Open University.

Gallagher, A. (2017) Care ethics and nursing practice (Chapter 15), in A. Scotts (eds) *Key Concepts and Issues in Nursing Ethics*. s.l., Springer Cham, pp. 55–68.

Gallagher, A. (2020) *Slow Ethics and the Art of Care*. Bingley: Emerald Publishing.

Gallagher, A. and Herbert, C. (2019) *Faith and Ethics in Health and Social Care: Improving Practice Through Understanding Diverse Faith Perspectives*. London and Philadelphia: Jessica Kingsley Publishers.

Gallagher, A., Naden, D. and Karterud, D. (2016) 'Ethical aspects of robots in care', *Nursing Ethics*, 23(4), pp. 369–371.

Gallagher, A., Peacock, M., Zasada, M., Coucke, T., Cox, A. and Janssens N. (2017) 'Care-givers' reflections on an ethics education immersive simulation care experience: A series of epiphanous events', *Nursing Inquiry*, 24(3), pp. 1–10.

Gallagher, A., Williams, E., Peacock, M., Zasada, M. and Cox, A. (2020) 'Findings from a mixed methods pragmatic cluster trial evaluating the impact of ethics education interventions on residential care-givers', *Nursing Inquiry*, 28 (2), pp. 1–12.

Gastmans, C. (1999) 'Care as A Moral Attitude in Nursing', *Nursing Ethics*, 6(3), pp. 214–223.

Gilligan, C. (1982) *In a Different Voice: Psychological Theory and Women's Development*. Cambridge, MA: Harvard University Press.

Gillon, R. (1986) *Philosophical Medical Ethics*. London: John Wiley and Sons.

Glassdoor (2021) 'Organisational culture and climate: what are the differences?' Available at: https://glassdoor.com/blog/guide/climate-vs-culture/ (Accessed 2 March 2023.

Haddad, L.M. and Geiger, R.A. (2022) *Nursing Ethical Considerations* [e-book]. Treasure Island, FL: StatPearls Publishing. Available at: www.ncbi.nlm.nih.gov/books/NBK526054/ (Accessed 10 March 2023).

Harper, S. J. (2009) 'Ethics versus morality: A problematic divide', *Philosophy & Social Criticism*, 35(9), pp. 1063–1077.

Haugen, I. (2020) 'Homesickness for people with dementia', in B. Pasveer, O. Synnes and I. Moser (eds), *Ways of Home Making in Care for Later Life*. Singapore: Palgrave Macmillan, pp. 65–84.

Honoré, C. (2005) *In Praise of Slowness: Challenging the Cult of Speed*. New York: Harper One.

Hunter, K. and Cook, C. (2018) 'Role-modelling and the hidden curriculum: New graduate nurses' professional socialisation', *Journal of Clinical Nursing*, 27(15–17), pp. 3157–3170.

International Council of Nurses (2021) *The ICN Code of Ethics for Nurses*. Geneva: International Council of Nurses. Available at: www.icn.ch/system/files/2021-10/ICN_Code-of-Ethics_EN_Web_0.pdf (Accessed 4 April 2023).

Johnstone, M. (2019) *Bioethics – A Nursing Perspective 8e*. 8th edn. Australia: Elsevier Health Sciences.

Johnstone, M. J. and Hutchinson, A. (2015) '"Moral distress" – Time to abandon a flawed nursing construct?' *Nursing Ethics*, 22(1), pp. 5–14.

Kamphof, I. and Hendriks, R. (2020) 'Beyond façade: home making and truthfulness in dementia care' in B, Pasveer, O. Synnes and I. Moser (eds) *Ways of Home Making in Care for Later Life*. Singapore: Palgrave Macmillan, pp. 271–292.

Kelly, S.H. (2020) 'The hidden curriculum: Undergraduate nursing students' perspectives of socialization and professionalism', *Nursing Ethics*, 27(5), pp. 1250–1260.

Koskenvuori, J., Stolt, M., Suhonen, R. and Leino-Kilpi, H. (2018) 'Healthcare professionals' ethical competence: A scoping review', *Wiley Nursing Open*, 6(1).

Learner, S. (2015) 'Therapeutic lying can be beneficial in dementia care but should "be used as a last resort"'. Available at: www.carehome.co.uk/news/article.cfm/id/1572600/therapeutic-lying-dementia-care (Accessed 26 April 2023)

Lechasseur, K., Caux, A., Dollé, S. and Legault, A. (2018) 'Ethical competence: An integrative review', *Nursing Ethics*, 25(6), pp. 694–706.

Lynch, D., Surdyk, P. and Eiser, A. (2004) 'Assessing professionalism: a review of the literature', *Medical Teacher*, 26(4), pp. 366–373.

McCarthy, J. and Gastmans, C. (2015) 'Moral distress: A review of the argument-based literature', *Nursing Ethics*, 22(1), pp. 131–152.

Mill, M.S. (1863) *Utilitarianism*. London: Parker, Son and Bourn.

Monteverde, S. (2014) 'Caring for tomorrow's workforce: Moral resilience and healthcare ethics education', *Nursing Ethics*, 23(1), pp. 104–116.

Noddings, N. (1984) *A Feminine Approach to Ethics and Moral Education*. Berkeley: University of California Press.

Nursing and Midwifery Council (2017) 'Enabling Professionalism in nursing and midwifery practice'. Available at: www.nmc.org.uk/globalassets/sitedocuments/other-publications/enabling-professionalism.pdf (Accessed 31/01/2023).

Nursing and Midwifery Council (2018) 'The code: standards of conduct, performance and ethics for nurses and midwives'. Available at: www.nmc.org.uk/globalassets/sitedocuments/nmc-publications/nmc-code.pdf (Accessed 31/01/2023).

Office of the Public Guardian (2014) 'Mental Capacity Act: making decisions' (www.gov.uk/government/collections/mental-capacity-act-making-decisions (Accessed 7th April 2023).

Online Etymology Dictionary. (no date) 'Ethics (n.)' [online]. Available at: www.etymonline.com/word/ethics (Accessed 2 April 2023).

Oxford English Dictionary (2022) 'profession, (n.)' [online]. Available at: www.oed.com/view/Entry/152052#eid28085893 (Accessed 31 January 2023).

Pauly, B., Varcoe, C., Storch, J. and Newton, L. (2009) 'Registered nurses' perceptions of moral distress and ethical climate', *Nursing Ethics*, 16 (5), pp. 561–573.

Rawling, P. (2023) *Deontology*. Cambridge: Cambridge University Press.

Revell, A. (2017) *Apartheid: A History of Apartheid,* s.l.: Independently Published.

Savulescu, J., Persson, I. and Wilkinson, D. (2020) 'Utilitarianism and the pandemic', *Bioethics*, 34(6), pp. 620–632.

Sevier, H. (2021) *Consequentialist Ethics: The Battle between Deontology and Consequentialism: The Trolley Problem*. s.l.: Independently Published.

Steinweis, A.E. and Rachlin, R.D. eds. (2013) *The Law in Nazi Germany: Ideology, Opportunism, and the Perversion of Justice*. New York: Berghahn.

Tuckett, A.G. (2004) 'Truth-telling in clinical practice and the arguments for and against: a review of the literature', *Nursing Ethics*, 11(5), pp. 500–513.

Wagner, P., Hendrich, J., Moseley, G. and Hudson, V. (2007) 'Defining medical professionalism: a qualitative study', *Medical Education*, 41, pp. 288–294.

Zingmark, K., Norbert, A. and Sandman, P-O. (1993) 'Experience of at homeness and homesickness in patients with Alzheimer's disease', *American Journal of Alzheimer's Care and Related Disorders & Research*, 8 (3), pp. 10–16.

4 Evidence for Nursing Practice Pillar

Kris Deering, Holly Sugg, Charli Morris, Malcolm Turner, Nikita Bailey, and Bel McDonald

Introduction

This chapter considers the meanings and roles of evidence in nursing practice, research, and nurse education. Specific lenses have shaped evidence-based practice (EBP) over the years, most notably detailing levels of evidence which place systematic reviews (methodical literature reviews of evidence), and meta-synthesis (statistical syntheses of findings from multiple studies) as gold standard research methodologies (Guyatt et al., 1995). However, in the context of nursing, evidence needs to be explored in relation to its utility to those accessing health and social care services. Adopting a pragmatist philosophy, we argued that evidence should be meaningful to the lives of those accessing and receiving care (Miller, Fins, and Bacchetta, 1996). As patient participation is a significant part of care practice and research, pragmatism sits well with exploring different forms of evidence, to ensure it is relevant to the needs of patients and their loved ones. While establishing the efficacy of interventions requires stringent research methodologies, such as randomised control trials (RCTs) (see below) these may not fully capture what it is like to live with a condition (Morgan, 2014). Hence, the concept of 'methodological congruence' will be considered, whereby the study aim dictates the research design, and the experiences and views of patients and their significant others are also important evidence bases.

This chapter commences with a scenario outlining how evidence concerning safety when nursing a patient with mental health needs might come in different forms. This is further debated in the section on pragmatism. An overview of the EBP pillar will follow, including a sketch of EBP within the nursing context. Thereafter, pragmatism will be explored in terms of its practical application to enhance the meaningfulness of evidence. Learning strategies, focused on methodological congruence will then be discussed, with a view to enriching student curiosity around critique of evidence and its utility in nursing practice. How evidence can be pluralistic and provisional in meeting the needs of the whole person during various times of accessing healthcare will be considered (Brendel, 2006). Key to this is how an awareness of fallibility, and willingness to challenge potentially incorrect assertions, aids exploring meaningful options for the patient. For that reason, the chapter will conclude with a consideration of reflective practices within evidence-based nursing (Dolan, Nowell, and Graham, 2022).

DOI: 10.4324/9781003390565-4

Scenario

Onisha is a 21-year-old woman who recently started to attend university. The difficulties of moving from home, alongside the pressures of university life, has contributed to Onisha drinking up to two bottles of wine per day. Onisha reached a crisis point when found unconscious by her roommate and taken to the local emergency department. Upon waking, Onisha said she felt unsafe and overwhelmed, stating that she had taken an overdose of paracetamol tablets. She struggled to explain the reasons for the overdose and, when asked if she would like support from friends and family, Onisha was reluctant to agree because she did not wish to 'hassle' people. Due to concerns about her mental health, Onisha was referred to the psychiatric liaison team based in the hospital, however, Onisha had to wait for this service due to the number of referrals that day.

Following the administration of intravenous fluids, the results of blood tests to assess Onisha's alcohol and paracetamol levels showed long-term alcohol use and a substantial paracetamol overdose, notably 'Paracetamol ingested at a dose greater than the licensed daily dose and more than or equal to 75 mg/kg [within] 24 hours' (Grundlingh and Ribeiro, 2023). The severity of the overdose raised concerns that Onisha may be at a greater risk of suicide than originally understood and that she may have downplayed the risk to avoid inconveniencing others. On this day, there was a higher degree of staff sickness and patient admissions to the department than usual. While Onisha spoke about gaining comfort from the nurses, they were only able to stay for short periods owing to the bustle of the department. Furthermore, according to some nurse views, Onisha needed to reduce her reliance on staff time to manage the increased patient admissions. Onisha noticed that the nurses decreased their time with her. Although a sedative was offered when physically safe to do so, Onisha interpreted this as being bothersome to others, as medication rather than nursing time was adopted to lessen Onisha's distress, raising fears around what might happen next with her care.

Evidence-Based Practice: Application to Nursing

The EBP pillar consists of wide-ranging concepts and practices to aid a person who, as in the above scenario, is experiencing some form of mental distress. Most importantly, evidence should help assist a patient's 'recovery', and as illustrated in Chapter 6, this is whereby a person is supported to have a meaningful life despite experiencing mental health difficulties (Anthony, 1993). Evidence ideally goes beyond theoretical or scientific knowledge, to include an understanding of patients' lived experiences, which enrich traditional expert knowledge with new perspectives (Honey et al., 2020). It is also complemented by values-based practice, as introduced in the previous chapter relating to evidence and professionalism. Before exploring these ideas, the chapter will summarise the development of EBP, including a brief history and the current application to nursing practice.

Brief History of EBP

EBP may be considered a relatively modern phenomenon, with evidence-based medicine (EBM) practices emerging in the 1970s (Guyatt, 1991), focusing on establishing the effectiveness of pharmacological treatments through conducting rigorous research (Smith and Rennie, 2014). Also, relatively recent are randomised controlled trials (RCTs) involving participants randomised to groups to compare treatments and limit biases, adopted in their modern form in the late 1940s, to improve the safety of medicine (Bothwell et al., 2016). The history of EBP, however, predates these developments with examples from Ancient Greece in which evidence disputed the existence of mythological Gods, to the Renaissance following the Middle Ages, with improving the investigating of human anatomy. Better known is Florence Nightingale, a nurse in the 1800s, who chronicled physical observations and developed statistical analysis to assess and improve patient care (Mackey and Bassendowski, 2017). However according to Durgun (2013), these examples suggest a Eurocentrism with determining evidence, particularly concerning health care, overlooking other valuable practices beyond Europe and from around the globe.

It is also argued that research ethics has progressed slower than EBP, with many instances of research ethics violations. Examples include the American Public Health Service syphilis study in Tuskegee (www.tuskegee.edu/about-us/centers-of-excellence/bioethics-center/about-the-usphs-syphilis-study) in which, between 1932 and 1972, African American men were recruited to the study without informed consent, without knowing their diagnosis, and they were not offered treatment for syphilis when this became available (see, for example, Gray, 1998). In modern times, substandard research has resulted in ethical ramifications, such as Wakefield's assertion that the MMR (measles, mumps, and rubella) vaccine caused childhood autism (Eggertson, 2010). This misleading evidence still influences fears about vaccines today and contributes to lower uptake, with significant impact on public health (Motta and Stecula, 2021).

Despite Guyatt not coining the term EBM until 1991, there are earlier examples of evaluating healthcare procedures. Notable is Archie Cochrane devising the first systematic review, initiating the Cochrane Systematic Review Library in the 1970s (Starr et al., 2009). Since then, the United Kingdom (UK) National Institute for Health and Care Excellence was formed in 1999, creating guidelines commonplace within international nursing. This, in part, was influenced by the Calman–Hine report (1995), criticising the expertise and accessibility of cancer services (Morris et al., 2008). In terms of nursing, it is suggested that EBP is influenced by the ideas of EBM which emphasises the conduct of rigorous research to inform technologies and treatments, to lessen iatrogenic risks (patient harms caused by interventions) (Lipscomb, 2016). This has resulted in some critique, in that what constitutes evidence in nursing can to an extent be shaped by views entrenched in EBM (Pitsillidou et al., 2021). According to Foucault (1980), such views may influence the prioritising of empirical evidence, focused on what is observable and measurable, not always accommodating the experiential knowledge of patients and what might be personally meaningful within their care (Williams and Garner, 2002).

Hierarchies of Evidence

While many hierarchies of evidence exist, in which research methodologies are ranked according to rigour, the hierarchy by Guyatt et al. (1995) remains somewhat a focal point for nurse education. It is important to recognise how providing one hierarchy without critique might impact on student learning, implying that following a specific hierarchy is the only method of determining quality evidence (Vere and Gibson, 2021). This appears especially problematic, given that Blunt (2015) identified 195 hierarchies around medicine alone, suggesting philosophical positions can help to shape what constitutes 'evidence'.

Philosophical views about evidence can be difficult to grasp, nevertheless, these positions inform our thinking in what can be seen as reality, situated around the topic of 'ontology' which involves assumptions about how we consider something to be real (Blaikie, 2000). For example, as discussed with pragmatism below, reality is determined by encompassing some usefulness to improving social difficulties (Bernstein, 1989), whereas other ontologies, notably objectivism, denote a fact-based and absolute world, and this can include how things work involving physiology, or the actions of gravity, in which reality is not something we can necessarily experience (Bryman, 2016). To understand reality, we require knowledge of ontology, and in a sense, this is enlightened by 'epistemology', surrounding the ways we come to know aspects of the world (Crotty, 1998). Although a fuller account is provided within the methodological congruence section, broadly, there are things we know that are not literally experienced, such as knowledge of a volcano without witnessing an eruption, while some suggest knowledge is only gained via our experiences (Lincoln, Lynham, and Guba, 2017).

Many philosophical positions exist, influencing how evidence is perceived and what methodologies are best suited to answer research questions. These determine whether, for example, a quantitative study or qualitative study is most relevant. Indeed, some philosophers question the need to even have such distinctions. Hence, in nurse education it could be suggested that understanding philosophical positions is necessary to appreciate different forms of evidence and methodologies, and to understand this further, these points are developed when discussing pragmatism and methodological congruence below.

Reflecting on the hierarchy by Guyatt et al. (1995), focus appears to be on researching pharmacological treatments, though suggests a wider healthcare application beyond medicine. Investigating medication undeniably requires the adoption of particular research methodologies, namely RCTs and meta-analysis of RCTs to establish effectiveness. Nevertheless, not all research questions relating to the enhancement of patient experience, can be responded to by an RCT, particularly when assisting with personalised mental health needs. More recent iterations of the hierarchy have emphasised expert opinion on the lowest rung as shown in Figure 4.1 (Hoffman, Bennett, and Del Mar, 2013). While, again, this may be suitable for certain treatments, it may not best inform patient 'recovery', which entails the experiences of patients and their loved ones in what aids a meaningful life (Slade, 2012).

Recently, there have been developments concerning the existence of many hierarchies, and although somewhat focused on medicine, the following concepts by Vere and Gibson (2021) can aid critical thinking around hierarchical application. Firstly, *professional jurisdiction* (asking 'what evidence informs practice') suggests that exploring patient experiences, for example, is an influential evidence base in nursing. Secondly, *practical concerns* relates to the practicalities of the profession in the work they do with patients. Thereafter, *methodological quality* is considered; however, this is difficult to determine without first understanding methodological congruence: the link between the study aim and research design. Thus, the 'quality' of evidence, and appropriateness of research methodologies, depends upon the purpose of the research. Indeed, research designs may be somewhat incomparable, depending on the study aim, similarly to a bike cannot be critiqued for going slower than a car, and a car cannot

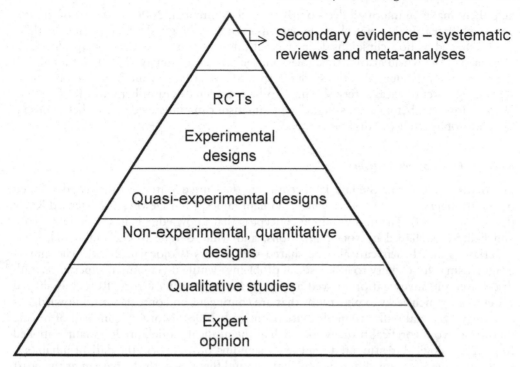

Figure 4.1 Hierarchy of evidence
Adapted from Schmidt and Brown (2021, p. 16)

be critiqued for being sedentary compared to the bike, as their purposes are different despite both defined as vehicles. Lastly, Vere and Gibson (2021) reflect the importance of methodological congruence in their acknowledgement of *different questions*, in that the aim of what is being explored impacts on what constitutes evidence. Hence, and shown in the following figures, knowledge of different methodologies and their purposes is a starting point for student learning. However, beforehand; an introduction to pragmatism is provided given its significance to addressing evidence in terms of patient care.

The Application of Pragmatism

It may appear that the scenario involving Onisha has so far been forgotten; yet its relevance to EBP will be explored in the context of pragmatism: a philosophy within which 'evidence' is perhaps less about determining 'truth', and more about having utility in aiding those with direct experience of the problem (Lamb, 2019). It is not the case that pragmatism simplifies evidence by seeking mere agreeability with those it concerns. Utility cannot be determined simply by experience; it involves an interplay of deductive and inductive reasoning termed abduction (Peirce, 1998 [1903]). As such, both objective views about the world, and how the world is subjectively experienced, are acknowledged (Peirce, 1998 [1903]).

Hypotheses from objective views are tested against patient experiences to assess relevance, requiring evidence to be translated in ways which resonate with the patient and help them make an informed decision (Burks, 1946; Brendel, 2006). In terms of the scenario, while reasonable that clinical concerns exist regarding risks such as suicide, these can be shaped by how clinicians define patient safety and may not fully encapsulate how Onisha sees the world at that time (Slemon, Jenkins, and Bungay, 2017). Although not their intention, the nurses' actions are interpreted via an impact on Onisha's self-worth, suggesting psychological safety should also be considered within her care (Burke et al., 2019). However, before discussing how pragmatism can guide evidence to help Onisha, the philosophy itself will first be outlined.

Relevant Tenets of Pragmatism

Pragmatism stems from the late 19th century in the United States of America, developed by philosophers such as Charles Peirce, William James, John Dewey, and Richard Rorty (Goodman, 1998). The underpinning concept is that knowledge is based on experience and beliefs, as shaped by social situations, and while unique to the individual, these experiences and beliefs can also be shared with others (Cojocaru, 2020). The aim of pragmatism is for enquiry to lessen social problems identified via human experience, with discussion and investigation viewed as crucial for minimising errors. Reality is shaped via enquiry which seeks explanations that are contingent on context, thus, knowledge is seen as provisional rather than absolute (Ormerod, 2006). Moreover, instead of relying on one or two theoretical frameworks such as the medical model, predominantly applied to pharmacological treatment, a joint understanding of the world the patient inhabits is built, allowing room for different explanations and theories with the patient at the heart of these accounts (Parascandola, Hawkins, and Danis, 2002). Hence, interpersonal relations and dialogue are necessary to understand such personal information, and with the scenario about Onisha, this appeared to not take place, leaving Onisha perhaps mistrustful about staff intentions.

Pragmatism makes space for plurality and fallibility, as the philosophy considers varying views in light that knowledge is ever-expanding and incorrect assertions of the world may be held (Marchetti, 2021). While patient views can seem unfamiliar perhaps due to mental health difficulties, these nevertheless matter and provide rich understanding about how care might be understood within the patient's own social context (Yung and Lin, 2016). To make sense of these views, understanding cannot be limited to preconceived boundaries of knowledge based on a few theoretical models. For example, although the reality that Onisha presents in the scenario may not align with the position held by the clinical team, particularly in terms of some abandonment, it is nonetheless Onisha's understanding of the world at that time, and meaningful within that time and space (Kendler, 2016). Hence, mutual grounds are sought whenever possible and however small, to improve the life of patients rather than create division about what constitutes 'truth', as 'the future is not determined [and] cooperating can make the world better' (Putnam, 2017, p. 111).

Clinical Pragmatism

The growth of pragmatism in the field of healthcare led to 'clinical pragmatism', drawing on the work of John Dewey (Brendel, 2006), a renowned educationalist who developed 'constructivism', in which learner experiences are viewed as enriching the meaningfulness of education (Dewey, 1896). Clinical pragmatism is applicable to mental health care, particularly resonating with recovery, whereby an evidence base is built around what is personally meaningful to the patient (Deering et al., 2021). This clinical orientation can assist Onisha on Practical, Plural, Participatory and Provisional grounds (Brendel, 2006). Questions arising from the scenario may include how any evidence is *practical* to Onisha's life, entailing an openness to a *pluralistic* reality in which (despite holding expertise) nurses question how the evidence resonates with Onisha, who may have different views (Brendel, 2006). With *participation*, Onisha's views go to the heart of her care. If unable to see the relevance, it might result in accusations of noncompliance by refusing the care provided, on the grounds that it appears immaterial or even harmful to Onisha's life (Brendel, 2006). Lastly, evidence is understood as *provisional*: whereby it is adapted to resonate with Onisha's views, thus context-driven to meet her needs in specific times and spaces (Brendel, 2006).

The challenge is when nurses ascribe particular ways of looking at the patient's world defined by a few intransigent concepts such as the medical model. Despite having a place in psychiatry with diagnosing and prescribing medicine, the medical model is critiqued as overly dominant with shaping care, and not the only concept that can aid patients such as Onisha (Allemang, Sitter, and Dimitropoulos, 2022). In the scenario, a primary nursing concern was mitigating risks like suicide. Despite Onisha somewhat sharing this view, other aspects concerning her safety might be overlooked when relying on one definition such as the medical model, in which deliberate self-harm tends to be assigned to mental illness (Slemon, Jenkins, and Bungay, 2017). Thus, considerations for iatrogenic psychological risks could go unnoticed. For example, Onisha is interpreting some nursing practices as a form of judgement. This might cultivate a negative self-image, increasing Onisha's distress of not seeing herself as a worthwhile person, and potentially contributing to her wanting to take her own life (Burke et al., 2019).

At times, the use of evidence may overly focus on patient outcomes, such as mitigating suicide, rather than the process of care. While outcomes are important, social connectivity to make sense of Onisha's world is also significant (Deering et al., 2021). Given that a sense of burdensomeness and thwarted belonging can be formulated around why people take their own lives, a social connectivity that Onisha is of worth might be beneficial in itself (Joiner, 2005). For example, asking more than once if Onisha can identify people meaningful to her, with a view to demonstrating that she is not a 'hassle' to others (Deering et al., 2019). This is supported by an objective evidence base yet in consideration of abduction, evidence is also shaped around the personal accounts of the patient.

Care can also be seen in terms of momentary periods relating to various times and spaces, with an understanding that a desire to live will not necessarily be a guaranteed outcome (Davidson, Tondora, and Ridgway, 2010). While the latter is ideal, 'care' may include many conversations to grasp how this objective is obtained. What can be more readily obtained, perhaps, is generating some ambivalence about suicide based on the value Onisha ascribes to her life. It is possible that a trauma going far back into her life contributes to her suicide risk (Ihme et al., 2022). Achieving desires to live might therefore take time, requiring nurses to sit with some uncertainty, especially while waiting for the psychiatric liaison team to respond. Hence how Onisha is helped to feel safe in such circumstances, beyond clinical risk concerns, is an important part of evidence gathering (Hunt et al., 2021).

While pragmatism can be unfairly accused of an incompatibility with some undisputable knowledge, it also proposes that diverse and contradictory perspectives of the world can coexist in various times and spaces (Colapietro, 1986). To avoid hampering the development of new and rich knowledge, we cannot merely assert that we know all there is to know (Putnam, 2017). With the above scenario, evidence informing care could be constructed around the world of the nurse. The complexity of the working environment and challenges of not being able to resolve difficulties quickly seem significant. However, if not investigated in context, such considerations may result in judgements around the patient, notably, taking up limited clinical time (O'Keeffe et al., 2021). Nonetheless, clinical decision-making may intersect with subjective understandings of the world at that time, and while issues may appear attributed to the patient, the evidence on how a busy working environment might shape decisions involving Onisha's care should not be overlooked (Roennfeldt et al., 2021).

The points raised highlight that framing evidence only via perceived absolutes can create obstacles to grasping what is helpful according to patient views which, like all humans, can vary in diverse times and spaces. To demonstrate, this section concludes with a thought experiment, intended to aid considering evidence in terms of its meaningfulness to life (note that the intention is not to endorse conspiracy theories, especially when these cause harm). Thus, if we were to suggest that the flat-earth theory is a legitimate scientific position, in which the world is believed flat, then the authors might be proverbially laughed out of the room. Yet, if behind the theory there exists a rich community of people who in the past felt estranged but are now embraced, then the experiment asks in what way does the 'truth' of the theory matter, and are the experiences of belongingness also an important part of evidence, with enriching a quality of life (Van Prooijen and Douglas, 2018)?

Methodological Congruence and Research Appraisal

Scrutinising research plays a significant role within nursing practice and education, given the expectation that nurses keep abreast of the latest research to inform their practice. Education, therefore, is important in developing critical thinking about research. However, the utility of such learning also requires consideration. There is little point in students engaging in research-related subjects if they lack the motivation and understanding to do so. Such motivation can be subjective and, in terms of nursing, can be driven by ethical positions (Vanlaere and Gastmans, 2007). Thus, returning to the role of values-based practice, motivation can be enriched via concepts such as social justice, involving equitable rights especially in fields where patients find this wanting (Hosseinzadegan, Jasemi, and Habibzadeh, 2021). Moreover, when considering Dewey's aforementioned constructivism, it is necessary to relate research to practices already experienced by students to render research less onerous in their eyes, as well as highlight its importance to practice. For example, data collection methods such as patient conversations and physical observations suggest that in some way students are already involved in research-related practices. To simply state, for example, that learning about research is required to qualify is a 'straw man' argument, as it lacks a buy in as to why students should, and despite much attention on lifelong learning in nursing, may even suggest keeping abreast of research is less needed when qualified.

Critiquing research papers perhaps requires an underlying reason that students can relate to around the value they give to the role of research to enhance nursing practice. Meanwhile, educators need some awareness of their own fallibility, such as inexperience

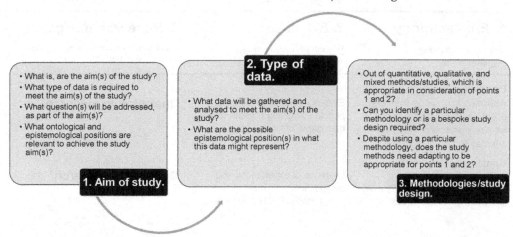

Figure 4.2 Process map of methodological congruence
Adapted from Saunders et al. (2019, p. 108)

around research approaches beyond their own field, so their preferred methodologies do not cloud student learning (Munby, 1982). All researchers hold preferences and ideals, but in terms of pragmatism, the role of an educator is not indoctrination to what they believe is correct. Rather, students should develop their own ideas, as can progress rich knowledge about the world (Schraw and Lori, 2003). To ensure parity among research methodologies, there is a growing trend to teach students about methodological congruence, involving understanding how the study aim, is informed, and informed by, ontological and epistemological stances, guiding the selection of a methodology (Willgens et al., 2016). That is, asking if the methodology is suitable to meet the study aim, rather than comparing different methodologies about what is best overall, as depends on what the study aimed to achieve. Accordingly, Figure 4.2 provides a potential guide for teaching methodological congruence.

Assessing methodological congruence requires knowledge of the purposes of nursing enquiry for, as previously outlined, the practice of the profession may link to the scope of the research, inclusive of the student's own ideas about the values underlying nursing practice, as highlighted in the ethics chapter, as well as above (Weaver and Olson, 2006). Thankfully, the research scope is broad in nursing, involving the lives of patients and significant others such as carers, including improving abilities to care informed by organisational knowledge, while investigating the wellbeing of nurses is also important, to name a few. Congruence, then, starts with an aim justifiable as nursing-related research, alongside knowledge in what way can the topic be investigated, informed by philosophical lenses, which also has bearing on the selection of methodology (Weaver and Olson, 2006).

While an extensive discussion of philosophy is beyond the parameters of this chapter, Figure 4.3 presents some explanations of philosophical lenses that may, but not absolutely, aid the selection of some research designs. For simplicity, designs are presented in terms of quantitative, qualitative, and mixed methods, as later outlined. Philosophical

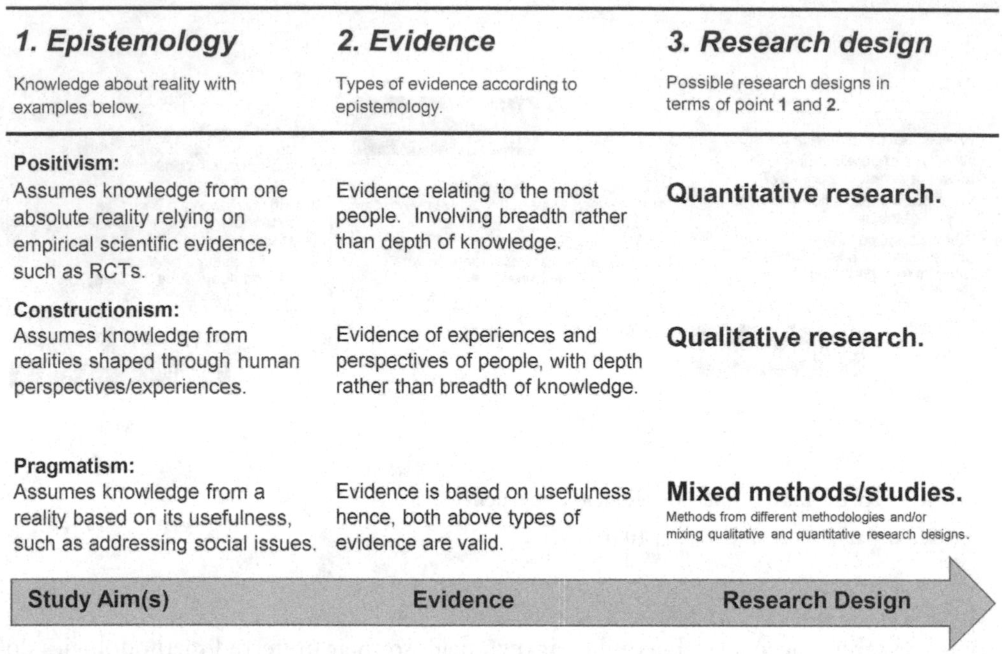

1. Epistemology	2. Evidence	3. Research design
Knowledge about reality with examples below.	Types of evidence according to epistemology.	Possible research designs in terms of point **1** and **2**.
Positivism: Assumes knowledge from one absolute reality relying on empirical scientific evidence, such as RCTs.	Evidence relating to the most people. Involving breadth rather than depth of knowledge.	**Quantitative research.**
Constructionism: Assumes knowledge from realities shaped through human perspectives/experiences.	Evidence of experiences and perspectives of people, with depth rather than breadth of knowledge.	**Qualitative research.**
Pragmatism: Assumes knowledge from a reality based on its usefulness, such as addressing social issues.	Evidence is based on usefulness hence, both above types of evidence are valid.	**Mixed methods/studies.** Methods from different methodologies and/or mixing qualitative and quantitative research designs.

Study Aim(s) — Evidence — Research Design →

Figure 4.3 Linking epistemology to evidence and research design
Adapted from Saunders et al. (2019, p. 108)

positions include assumptions made about the world involving beliefs and values, alongside ontological and epistemological stances, which inform the roadmap of the study design to meet particular research aims (Thurston, Cove, and Meadows, 2008). Despite aspirations to capture an objective reality in which the researcher is neutral (as per quantitative approaches), relationality to a design can be subjective. For example, which statistical measure to apply is somewhat interpretative, with the researcher's view determining the selection of research methods (Visser et al., 2022). While methods and methodology might be terms employed interchangeably, it is helpful to think of a distinction, whereby methodologies concern the overall research design, and methods are the steps to achieve the research (James, 2012). This is with the caveat that bespoke research designs can be devised to meet particular study aims and research questions, not necessarily fitting a standardised methodology.

Figure 4.3 shows why research designs might be adopted, contingent on epistemology and types of evidence. Quantitative methods tend to consider evidence with breadth and in numerical form, as important to test the efficacy of medicine for example, alongside grasping relationships between variables, such as disease within particular populations. Qualitative research involves smaller samples of detailed perspectives about the world, gathered via interviews for example, with non-numerical evidence such as words, photography, and film. Mixed methods/studies consist of methods from different methodologies, and/or mixing qualitative and quantitative approaches to gain a better insight into a topic (Morgan, 2014). While acknowledging this overview is broad, it is also somewhat purposeful. Providing examples of which standardised methodology may link to which epistemology can aid students in developing their own philosophical positions, and enrich critical thinking when evaluating research, in terms of what students see as personally meaningful about nursing practices. In addition, established critiquing tools are available, and the frameworks provided by Holland and Rees (2016) can help guide novices in asking in-depth questions for critiquing qualitative and quantitative research, accessible via a link within the reference list at the end of the chapter.

When critiquing quantitative research, *validity* is also considered: whether the outcome measures align with the study aim(s) and whether the findings reflect the population under study, alongside *reliability*: whether the results would be repeated using the same research methods in the same circumstances (Heale and Twycross, 2015). Given that the aims of qualitative research are different, *trustworthiness*, as first devised by Lincoln and Guba (1985), might instead be adopted. This involves assessing *credibility*: whether the study design can achieve the study aim(s) and whether the sample shares the experiences to be explored; *transferability*: whether the findings can be applied to other contexts, situations, times, and populations; *dependability*: whether enough methodological information is presented to enable critique; and *confirmability*: whether potential biases in the research have been addressed (Shenton, 2004). In terms of critiquing mixed methods/studies, the *Mixed Methods Appraisal Tool* by Hong, Gonzalez-Reyes and Pluye (2018) provides a useful starting point, and the link to their work is also available in the reference list.

Epistemologies and study aim(s), also shape questions aligning to what is intended to be explored. It can seem unnerving when considering the flexibility with devising research questions, and to lessen uncertainty, the use of memetic acronyms or initials to devise questions are recommended. PICO and PEO are suitable options, for quantitative and qualitative projects respectfully, relating to questions for research and literature reviews. PICO stands for what *population* aims to be explored, as well as what *intervention(s)*, while *comparison* involves comparing interventions, regarding the effectiveness between each other, concluding with their *outcome(s)* for the population (Butler, Hall, and Copnell, 2016). Hence this might involve exploring specific health interventions, with comparing the outcomes assessed by reducing symptoms of some kind, for a population. Alternatively, PEO can be more fitting for qualitative related projects, as less specific, allowing more flexibility to explore what is going on. Again, PEO involves a particular *population*, *exposure(s)* to something impacting that population, concluding on exploring the *outcome(s)* of the exposure, such as in terms of experiences and perspectives (Butler, Hall, and Copnell, 2016).

Reflectivity

Less explored within EBP is the use of reflection, first illustrated in the fundamentals of care chapter. It is a practice integral to nursing practice and education to improve care and challenge preconceived views which may cause harm. There is debate what 'reflection' means in the context of EBP, as evidence in care may be different to research evidence (Rycroft-Malone *et al.*, 2004). However, this chapter takes the position that there is little distinction, advocating for evidence to be as wide-ranging as needed to help others. This is a pragmatic concern whereby knowledge is ever-expanding; in addition, when responsible for others, an obligation exists to assess the relevance of evidence, and with nursing, this is to meet the needs of patients and their loved ones (Dolan, Nowell, and Graham, 2022). Reflection may centre on genuineness: understanding that, like all humans, one can be fallible, with cultivating different views in dialogue with others to generate an open-mindedness about what constitutes evidence when providing care (Deering, 2014). As such group supervision can be suitable, adopting a framework which allows safe consideration of other perspectives. The ladder of inference by Argyris and Schön (1974) is such a framework from the learning organisation literature, in which nurturing knowledge is embedded as part of a thriving organisational culture, touched upon in the ethics chapter (Tompkins and Rhodes, 2012).

As per Figure 4.4 below, beliefs and meanings, as influenced perhaps by the busy emergency department in the scenario, may shape conclusions. Conclusions could be

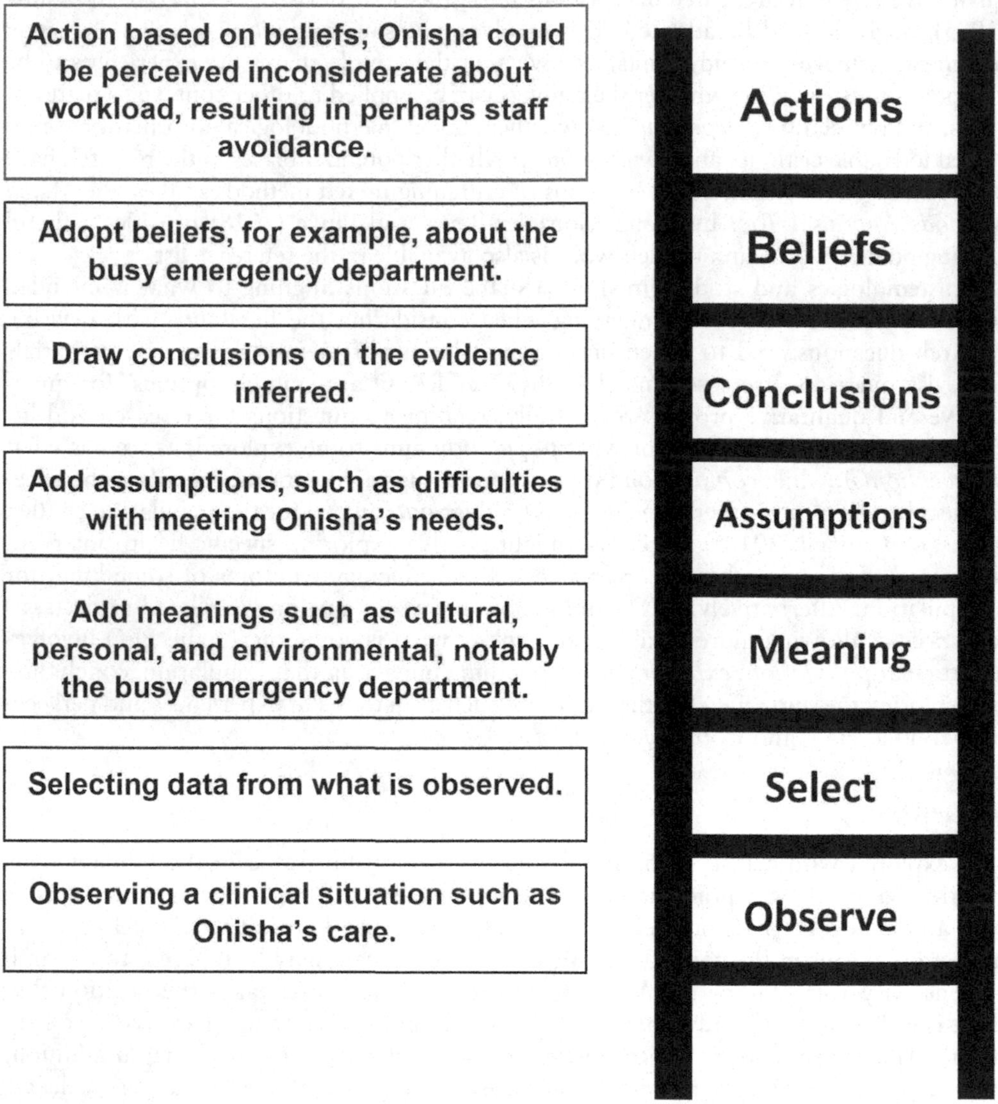

Figure 4.4 The ladder of inference
Adapted from Senge et al. (1994, p. 243)

drawn on many factors, but an awareness is needed that while noteworthy to the nurse and a potential influence on care, some factors might have little relevance to the patient. When discussed in a group, reflection may enable a considerate exploration around evidence in what the patient might find helpful (Cary and Marques, 2007). An overreliance on looking at the world via particular lenses can easily become entrenched, with evidence turning into something constituted through practices performed the same way for many years. Thus, consideration should be given to the notion that, despite appearing significant at the time, the evidence adopted in shaping care might be less valuable to those people who nurses ultimately serve, namely the patients and their loved ones (Deering, 2014).

Conclusion

This chapter outlined the EBP Pillar in terms of how nurses can work with evidence, expanding the EBP discussion beyond specific hierarchies and debates about which research methodologies are 'best'. Instead, the focus was on the utility of evidence as a means of helping patients, particularly when experiencing mental distress. Possible interventions, and evidence of their effectiveness, were deliberately avoided in discussing the case study, as without first understanding Onisha's views, the meaningfulness of such evidence is yet to be known. Thus, questions were instead posed to expand what might constitute evidence to help Onisha. Motivating student interest in research and encouraging critical thinking about methodological congruence, alongside utilising reflective practices, were also outlined. Essentially, one type of evidence cannot be seen as better than another without considering the needs of the patient and their loved ones. Nurses, regardless of knowledge and position, cannot determine what always constitutes the best evidence for everyone, owing to the diversity with which the world is viewed in various times and spaces. Hence, an openness to fallibility and humility can be helpful, to broaden an inclusiveness of different perspectives in what evidence might entail.

Takeaways for Student Nurses

- The ideas of evidence-based medicine, and the 'hierarchy of evidence', are important for informing evidence-based nursing practice. However, there is more than one way of deciding what constitutes the 'best' evidence for patients.
- Considering the needs and views of specific patients and their loved ones informs which type of evidence is 'best' for helping patients. The philosophical position of 'pragmatism' can help us build an evidence-base for patients around what is personally meaningful for them.
- Different research designs, such as quantitative, qualitative, and mixed method approaches, may be adopted depending on the study aim and our philosophical position(s). Thinking in terms of 'methodological congruence', or matching the methodology to the study purpose, therefore helps us decide which methodology is 'best'.

- As nurses should keep abreast of the latest research to inform their practice, scrutinising research is important. Focusing on methodological congruence and how different research designs link to different philosophical approaches can help critical thinking around evidence and its relevance for patients.
- It is important to remember that our knowledge and evidence may be wrong and changes over different times and spaces. Being reflective and considering different perspectives in evaluating evidence helps us to determine its applicability to specific patients.

Takeaways for Educators/Practitioners

- Evidence-based nursing practice is influenced by evidence-based medicine which prioritises empirical, observable and measurable evidence. However, providing only one hierarchy of evidence to students implies that there is only one method of determining quality evidence.
- Evidence should be considered in terms of its meaningfulness and utility to those accessing health and social care services. Pragmatism, involving an interplay of deductive and inductive reasoning, provides a lens through which to determine the relevance of evidence for patients.
- Rather than thinking in terms of evidence hierarchies alone, teaching 'methodological congruence' can ensure parity among research designs, such as quantitative, qualitative and mixed method approaches. As such, different philosophical positions influence how evidence is perceived, and the study aim guides the selection of the 'best' methodology.
- It is important to motivate students' critical thinking and interest in research. This can be enriched by relating research to practices experienced by students, providing examples of how different research designs link to different philosophical positions, and highlighting the value of research in enhancing nursing practice.
- Educators should avoid allowing their preferred or familiar methodologies to cloud student learning. An awareness of the fallibility and provisional nature of evidence, as well as engaging in group reflective processes which allow the safe consideration of different perspectives, can aid students to evaluate evidence.

References

Allemang, B., Sitter, K. and Dimitropoulos, G. (2022) 'Pragmatism as a paradigm for patient-oriented research', *Health Expectation*, 25(1), pp. 38–47.

Anthony, W. A. (1993) 'Recovery from mental illness: The guiding vision of the mental health service system in the 1990s', *Psychosocial Rehabilitation Journal*, 16(4), pp. 11–23.

Argyris, C. and Schön, D. A. (1974) *Theory in Practice: Increasing Professional Effectiveness.* California: Jossey-Bass Publishers.

Bernstein, R. J. (1989) 'Pragmatism, pluralism and the healing of wounds', *Proceedings and addresses of the American Philosophical Association*, 63(3), pp. 5–18.

Blaikie, N. (2000) *Designing Social Research*. Cambridge: Polity Press.

Blunt, C. (2015) *Hierarchies of Evidence in Evidence-Based Medicine*. PhD thesis, London School of Economics and Political Science. Available at: http://etheses.lse.ac.uk/3284/ (Accessed: 12 December 2022).

Bothwell, L.E., Greene, J.A., Podolsky, S.H. and Jones, D.S. (2016) 'Assessing the gold standard – lessons from the history of RCTs', *New England Journal of Medicine*, 374(22), pp. 2175–2181.

Brendel, H.B. (2006) *Healing Psychiatry: Bridging the Science/Humanism Divide*. London: The MIT Press.

Bryman, A. (2016) *Social Research Methods*. Oxford: Oxford University Press.

Burke, T.A., Piccirillo, M.L., Moore-Berg, S.L., Alloy, L.B. and Heimberg, R.G. (2019) 'The stigmatization of nonsuicidal self-injury', *Journal of Clinical Psychology*, 75(3) pp. 481–498.

Burks, A. W. (1946) 'Peirce's theory of abduction', *Philosophy of Science*, 13(4), pp. 301–306.

Butler, A., Hall, H. and Copnell, B. (2016) 'A guide to writing a qualitative systematic review protocol to enhance evidence-based practice in nursing and health care', *Worldviews on Evidence-Based Nursing*, 13(3), pp. 241–249.

Calman–Hine Report (1995) *A Report by the Expert Advisory Group on Cancer to the Chief Medical Officers of England and Wales. A Policy Framework for Commissioning Cancer Services – The Calman–Hine Report*. London: Department of Health.

Cary, D. and Marques, P. (2007) 'From expert to collaborator: Developing cultural competency in clinical supervision', *The Clinical Supervisor*, 26(1–2), pp. 141–157.

Cojocaru, M, D. (2020) 'Doing ethics or changing for the better? On pragmatism, ethics, and moral pragmatics', *Metaphilosophy*, 51(1) pp. 32–50.

Colapietro, V.M. (1986) 'William James's pragmatic commitment to absolute truth', *The Southern Journal of Philosophy*, 24(2), pp. 189–200.

Crotty, M. (1998) *The Foundations of Social Research: Meaning and Perspective in the Research Process*. London: SAGE.

Davidson, L., Tondora, J. and Ridgway, P. (2010) 'Life is not an "outcome": Reflections on recovery as an outcome and as a process', *American Journal of Psychiatric Rehabilitation*, 13(1), pp. 1–8.

Deering, K. (2014) 'Why doesn't the client listen to me? Challenging ethnocentricities through clinical supervision to promote cultural competencies', *Mental Health Nursing*, 34(6), pp. 10–12.

Deering, K., Pawson, C., Summers, N. and Williams, J. (2019) 'Patient perspectives of helpful risk management practices within mental health services. A mixed studies systematic review of primary research', *Journal of Psychiatric and Mental Health Nursing*, 26(5–6), pp. 185–197.

Deering, K., Williams, J., Stayner, K. and Pawson, C. (2021) 'Giving a voice to patient experiences through the insights of pragmatism', *Nursing Philosophy*, 22(1), online. Available at: https://onlinelibrary.wiley.com/doi/full/10.1111/nup.12329 (Accessed: 29 January 2023).

Dewey, J. (1896) 'The reflex arc concept in psychology', *Psychological Review*, 3(4), pp. 357–370.

Dolan, S., Nowell, L. and McCaffrey, G. (2022) 'Pragmatism as a philosophical foundation to integrate education, practice, research, and policy across the nursing profession', *Journal of Advanced Nursing*, 78(10), pp. 1–11.

Durgun, F. (2013) 'The idea of the progress, periodisation and the perception of medieval European history from the Renaissance to the 19th Century in European historiography', *Insan and Toplum Dergisi*, 3(6), pp. 283–304.

Eggertson, L. (2010) 'Lancet retracts 12-year-old article linking autism to MMR vaccines', *Canadian Medical Association Journal*, 182(4), pp. E199–200.

Foucault, M. (1980) *Power/Knowledge: Selected Interviews and Other Writings 1972–1977*. New York: Pantheon.

Goodman, R.B. (1998) 'Wittgenstein and pragmatism', *Parallax*, 4(4), pp. 91–105.

Gray, F.D. (1998) *The Tuskegee Syphilis Study: The Real Story and Beyond*. Montgomery, AL: NewSouth Books.

Grundlingh, J. and Ribeiro, C. (2023) 'BMJ best practice: Paracetamol overdose in adults'. Available at; https://bestpractice.bmj.com/topics/en-gb/3000110#:~:text=Serious%20toxicity%20 may%20occur%20in,in%20any%2024-hour%20per (Accessed: 1 March 2023).

Guyatt, G.H. (1991) 'Evidence-based medicine'. Available at: www.jameslindlibrary.org/guyatt-gh-1991/ (Accessed: 1 December 2022).

Guyatt, G.H., Sackett, D.L., Sinclair, J.C., Hayward, R., Cook, D.J., Cook, R.J., Bass, E., Gerstein, H., Haynes, B., Holbrook, A. and Jaeschke, R. (1995) 'Users' guides to the medical literature: IX. A method for grading health care recommendations', *Jama*, 274(22), pp. 1800–1804.

Heale, R. and Twycross, A. (2015) 'Validity and reliability in quantitative studies', *Evidence-based nursing*, 18(3), pp. 66–67.

Hoffmann, T., Bennett, S. and Del Mar, C.B. (2013) *Evidence-Based Practice across the Health Professions*. [e-book]. Elsevier Health Sciences. Available at: www.elsevier.com/books/evidence-based-practice-across-the-health-professions/hoffmann/978-0-7295-4255-5 (Accessed: 2 December 2022).

Holland, K. and Rees, C. (2016) 'Frameworks for critiquing research articles'. Available at: https:// global.oup.com/uk/orc/nursing/holland/01student/chapters/ch07/frameworks/ (Accessed 12 December 2022).

Honey, Boydell, K. M., Coniglio, F., Do, T. T., Dunn, L., Gill, K., Glover, H., Hines, M., Scanlan, J. N., and Tooth, B. (2020) Lived experience research as a resource for recovery: a mixed methods study. *BMC Psychiatry*, 20(1). Available at: https://bmcpsychiatry.biomedcentral.com/ articles/10.1186/s12888-020-02861-0 (Accessed: 3 January 2023).

Hong, Q. N., Gonzalez-Reyes, A. and Pluye, P (2018) 'Improving the usefulness of a tool for appraising the quality of qualitative, quantitative and mixed methods studies, the Mixed Methods Appraisal Tool (MMAT)', *Journal of Evaluation in Clinical Practice*, 24(3), pp. 459–467. Also available at: http://mixedmethodsappraisaltoolpublic.pbworks.com/w/file/fetch/127916259/ MMAT_2018_criteria-manual_2018-08-01_ENG.pdf (Accessed 29 January 2023).

Hosseinzadegan, F., Jasemi, M. and Habibzadeh, H. (2021) 'Factors affecting nurses' impact on social justice in the health system', *Nursing Ethics*, 28(1), pp. 118–130.

Hunt, D.F., Bailey, J., Lennox, B.R., Crofts, M. and Vincent, C. (2021) 'Enhancing psychological safety in mental health services', *International Journal of Mental Health Systems*, 15(1), pp. 1–18.

Ihme, Olié, E., Courtet, P., El-Hage, W., Zendjidjian, X., Mazzola-Pomietto, P., Consoloni, J.-L., Deruelle, C., and Belzeaux, R. (2022) 'Childhood trauma increases vulnerability to attempt suicide in adulthood through avoidant attachment', *Comprehensive Psychiatry*, 117, pp. 152,333–152,333.

James, A. (2012) *Research Methods and Methodologies in Education*. London: SAGE.

Joiner, T.E. (2005) *Why People Die by Suicide*. Cambridge, MA: Harvard University Press.

Kendler, K.S. (2016) 'The nature of psychiatric disorders', *World Psychiatry*, 15(1), pp. 5–12.

Lamb, R. (2019) 'Pragmatism, practices, and human rights', *Review of International Studies*, 45(4), pp. 550–568.

Lincoln, Y.S., Lynham, S.A. and Guba, E.G. (2017) 'Paradigmatic controversies, contradictions, and emerging influences, revisited', in N.K. Denzin and Y.S. Lincoln (eds), *The SAGE Handbook of Qualitative Research*, 5th edition. London: SAGE Publications, pp. 108–150.

Lincoln, Y.S. and Guba, E.G. (1985) *Naturalistic Inquiry*. Newbury Park, CA: Sage Publications.

Lipscomb, M. (2016) *Exploring Evidence-Based Practice: Debates and Challenges in Nursing. Routledge Key Themes in Health and Society*. London: Routledge.

Mackey, A. and Bassendowski, S. (2017) 'The history of evidence-based practice in nursing education and practice', *Journal of Professional Nursing*, 33(1), pp. 51–55.

Marchetti, S. (2021) *Introduction to Pragmatist Ethics: Theory and Practice. European Journal of Pragmatism and American Philosophy 13 (XIII-2)*. Available at: https://journals.openedition. org/ejpap/2664?lang=en (Accessed: 29 January 2023).

Miller, F.G., Fins J.J. and Bacchetta M.D. (1996) 'Clinical pragmatism: John Dewey and clinical ethics', *Journal of Contemporary Health Law and Policy*, 13, pp. 27–51.

Morgan, D. L. (2014) *Integrating Qualitative and Quantitative Methods: A Pragmatic Approach*. London: SAGE Publications.

Morris, E., Haward, R.A., Gilthorpe, M.S., Craigs, C. and Forman, D. (2008) 'The impact of the Calman-Hine report on the processes and outcomes of care for Yorkshire's breast cancer patients', *Annals of Oncology*, 19(2), pp. 284–291.

Motta, M. and Stecula, D. (2021) 'Quantifying the effect of Wakefield et al. (1998) on skepticism about MMR vaccine safety in the U.S', *PLoS ONE*, 16(8). Available at: https://journals.plos.org/plosone/article?id=10.1371/journal.pone.0256395 (Accessed: 29 January 2023).

Munby, H. (1982) 'The place of teachers' beliefs in research on teacher thinking and decision making, and an alternative methodology', *Instructional Science*, 11(3), pp. 201–225.

O'Keeffe, S., Suzuki, M., Ryan, M., Hunter, J. and McCabe, R. (2021) 'Experiences of care for self-harm in the emergency department: comparison of the perspectives of patients, carers and practitioners', *BJPsych Open*, 7(5), pp. 1–9.

Ormerod, R. (2006) 'The history and ideas of pragmatism', *Journal of the Operational Research Society*, 57(8), pp. 892–909.

Parascandola, M., Hawkins, J. and Danis. M. (2002) 'Patient autonomy and the challenge of clinical uncertainty', *Kennedy Institute of Ethics Journal*, 12, pp. 245–264.

Peirce, C.S. (1903/1998) 'Pragmatism as the logic of abduction', In The Peirce Edition Project (ed.), *The Essential Peirce: Selected Philosophical Writings, Volume II*. Bloomington, IN: Indiana University Press, pp. 1893–1913.

Pitsillidou, M., Roupa, Z., Farmakas, A. and Noula, M. (2021) 'Factors affecting the application and implementation of evidence-based practice in nursing', *Acta Informatica Medica*, 29(4), pp. 281–287.

Putnam, R.A. (2017) 'Reflections on the future of pragmatism', in D. Macarther (ed.), *Pragmatism as a Way of Life*. Cambridge, MA: Harvard University Press, pp. 108–123.

Roennfeldt, H., Wyder, M., Byrne, L., Hill, N., Randall, R. and Hamilton, B. (2021) 'Subjective experiences of mental health crisis care in emergency departments: A narrative review of the qualitative literature', *International Journal of Environmental Research and Public Health*, 18(18), pp. 1–22.

Rycroft-Malone, J., Seers, K., Titchen, A., Harvey, G., Kitson, A. and McCormack, B. (2004) 'What counts as evidence in evidence-based practice?', *Journal of Advanced Nursing*, 47(1), pp. 81–90.

Saunders, M., Lewis, P. and Thornhill, A. (2019) *Research Methods for Business Students*. New York: Pearson Education.

Schmidt, N.A. and Brown, J.M. (2021) *Evidence-Based Practice for Nurses: Appraisal and Application of Research*. Burlington MA: Jones and Bartlett Learning.

Schraw, G. and Olafson, L. (2003) 'Teachers' epistemological world views and educational practices', *Journal of Cognitive Education and Psychology*, 3(2), pp. 178–235.

Senge, P.M., Kleiner, A., Roberts, C., Ross, R.B. and Smith, B.J. (1994) *The Fifth Discipline Field Book*. New York: Doubleday.

Shenton, A.K. (2004) 'Strategies for Ensuring Trustworthiness in Qualitative Research Projects', *Education for Information*, 22, pp. 63–75. Also available at: www.pm.lth.se/fileadmin/_migrated/content_uploads/Shenton_Trustworthiness.pdf (Accessed: 29 January 2023).

Slade, M. (2012) 'The epistemological basis of personal recovery', in A. Rudnick (ed.), Recovery of People with Mental Illness: *Philosophical and Related Perspectives*. Oxford: Oxford University Press, pp. 78–92.

Slemon, A., Jenkins, E. and Bungay, V. (2017) 'Safety in psychiatric inpatient care: The impact of risk management culture on mental health nursing practice', *Nursing Inquiry*, 24(4), pp. 1–10.

Smith, R. and Rennie, D. (2014) 'Evidence-based medicine—an oral history', *Jama*, 311(4), pp. 365–367.

Starr, M., Chalmers, I., Clarke, M. and Oxman, A.D. (2009) 'The origins, evolution, and future of The Cochrane Database of Systematic Reviews', *International Journal of Technology Assessment in Health Care*, 25(S1), pp. 182–195.

Thurston, W.E., Cove, L. and Meadows, L.M. (2008) 'Methodological congruence in complex and collaborative mixed method studies', *International Journal of Multiple Research Approaches*, 2(1), pp. 2–14.

Tompkins, T.C. and Rhodes, K. (2012) 'Groupthink and the ladder of inference: Increasing effective decision making', *The Journal of Human Resource and Adult Learning*, 8(2), pp. 84–90.

Van Prooijen, J.W. and Douglas, K.M. (2018) 'Belief in conspiracy theories: Basic principles of an emerging research domain', *European Journal of Social Psychology*, 48(7), pp. 897–908.

Vanlaere, L. and Gastmans, C. (2007) 'Ethics in nursing education: learning to reflect on care practices', *Nursing Ethics*, 14(6), pp. 58–766.

Vere, J. and Gibson, B. (2021) 'Variation amongst hierarchies of evidence', *Journal of Evaluation in Clinical Practice*, 27(3), pp. 624–630.

Visser, L.N., van der Velden, N.C., Smets, E.M., van der Lelie, S., Nieuwenbroek, E., van Vliet, L.M. and Hillen, M.A. (2022) 'Methodological choices in experimental research on medical communication using vignettes: The impact of gender congruence and vignette modality', *Patient Education and Counseling*, 105(6), pp. 1634–1641.

Weaver, K. and Olson, J.K. (2006) 'Understanding paradigms used for nursing research', *Journal of Advanced Nursing*, 53(4), pp. 459–469.

Willgens, A.M., Cooper, R., Jadotte, D., Lilyea, B., Langtiw, C.L. and Obenchain-Leeson, A., (2016) 'How to enhance qualitative research appraisal: Development of the methodological congruence instrument', *The Qualitative Report*, 21(12), pp. 2380–2395.

Williams, D.D.R. and Garner, J. (2002) 'The case against 'the evidence': a different perspective on evidence-based medicine', *The British Journal of Psychiatry*, 180(1), pp. 8–12.

Yung, A.R. and Lin, A. (2016) 'Psychotic experiences and their significance', *World Psychiatry*, 15(2), pp. 130–131.

5 Patient and Public Involvement Pillar

Marie Clancy, Ana Maria Gomez Corrales,
Bethany Gooding, and Bel McDonald

Introduction

Patient and public involvement (PPI) is defined by the National Institute for Health Research (NIHR) as research being carried out 'with' or 'by' members of the public rather than 'to', 'about', or 'for' them (INVOLVE, 2013). However, the activities of PPI groups in universities go beyond research and also include contributions to learning and teaching, to scholarship and to curriculum development. This chapter considers how student and registered nurses work in partnership with patients, family members, informal caregivers, and members of PPI groups upholding the principle of 'nothing about us without us' (Charlton, 2000). In order to work effectively with PPI members, nurses need to listen to and learn from the patient voice, so patients and their significant others have an active role in the process of health and social care decision-making.

Patient and public involvement has become an integral part of health and social care research and education with its focus on including and empowering patients and the public in the shaping of care services (Mockford et al., 2012). However, this has not always been the case. Movement towards an open, patient-centred service to establish patients' involvement in health care services started in the 1950s (Entwistle et al., 1998). At this time, there was an assumption that medical practitioners were the only experts, and their opinions and authority could or should not be questioned (Charlton, 2000). The public began to challenge this as their disappointment and dissatisfaction with the health service increased. This was precipitated by an awareness that the views and perspectives of individuals and communities were not included or valued in decisions made about their health (Wilson et al., 2015).

While the PPI terrain is broad, this chapter will focus on a family scenario, demonstrating the importance of collaborative communication. The chapter explores how to include the patient voice, as well as their significant others, cultivating a care package that resonates with their needs, while also touching on how their experiences can inform nurse education. This is while the expertise of people, such as the family represented, informs their care. Drawing on relevant experiences the education section will utilise, among others, student nurse perspectives and how learning enriches awareness of care needs.

The chapter will conclude by adopting PPI perspectives within research ensuring, whenever possible, that participation is an equal partnership between researchers and PPI members. The focus on the child of the family in the anonymised scenario, also explores how children and young people's perspectives are understood, whether as research partners, education providers or patients with their perspectives also shaping nursing care.

DOI: 10.4324/9781003390565-5

To ensure the consolidation of learning, this chapter brings together pertinent reflective points to summarise each section, taking into consideration the complexity and value of enriching authentic participation with PPI group members. This is while these points are summarised concluding the chapter, alongside providing links to media outputs drawing on living experiences about the importance of PPI.

Scenario

Naajy is a 10-year-old refugee from Syria, who has been in the UK with his family for the last four years. Naajy was born by emergency caesarean section due to foetal distress. He required prolonged resuscitation at birth and active treatment as he experienced hypoxic ischaemic encephalopathy (HIE), a type of brain injury resulting from a lack of oxygen to the brain during the neonatal period which can cause life-long morbidity and premature mortality (Greco et al., 2020; Adstamongkonkul and Hess, 2017). Naajy has cerebral palsy, complex epilepsy and learning disabilities. Since arriving in the United Kingdom (UK), he is well known to the multidisciplinary team, with his condition deemed life-limiting or palliative. Children with palliative care needs have a primary, multifaceted, life-limiting or life-threatening condition. Life-limiting conditions (LLC) are said to have no reasonable hope of cure and children will die as a result. Life-threatening conditions (LTC), have viable, curative treatment but this may not always be successful (Thompson, 2015).

Naajy and his family are isolated and have very little social support, having left all their family and support networks following the conflict in Syria. Naajy has 18-month-old twin siblings, who he adores. His mum, Farah, is Naajy's full-time carer and also looks after his siblings at home. His father, Ibrahim, works night shifts in a factory and is limited in his ability to support Farah with caring responsibilities. The family also struggle financially and live in a small inaccessible flat. They are on the housing waiting list and this is a source of great anxiety for them. Naajy attends a special education school where he receives physiotherapy and speech and language therapy. His family also access the support of a learning disability nurse, as needed. Naajy has regular paediatrician, orthopaedic and specialist epilepsy appointments, which his family sometimes struggle to attend. He is learning Makaton to help him communicate.

Application of Patient and Public Involvement Pillar to Scenario

Our aims are to engage with the scenario of Naajy and his family, to detail each of the areas below with a focus on creativity and to propose approaches to meet the family's needs. By doing so, the chapter will address pertinent PPI aspects such as location of care, listening and communication.

Nursing Practice

Striving to maintain and improve quality of care for patients and families should be an 'intrinsic part of everyone's job every day, in all parts of the system' (Batalden and

Davidoff, 2007, p. 2). An important indicator for measuring the quality of service in health and social care is patient experience, with increasing evidence that such experience is positively associated with clinical effectiveness and patient safety (Department of Health and Social Care, 2012). Therefore, in addition to focusing on clinical outcomes, measuring patient satisfaction is essential to improving patient-centred care (Institute of Medicine, 2001; Jensen et al., 2016).

Involvement of patients and carers, in the improvement of services, offers opportunities to discover what really makes a difference to their experience and provides a better understanding of their needs and priorities. Subsequently, working in partnership with patients and carers can lead to increased staff morale as they can provide the care which is required, and requested, by the patients rather than assumed by clinicians (Jensen et al., 2016; Tallentire, Harley, and Watson, 2019; Smith, Hicks, and McGovern, 2020).

Naajy has been admitted to hospital with a bone infection, which requires long term intravenous antibiotic therapy (IVAB). The family wishes to receive the treatment at home where they feel safe, following the trauma they experienced during the conflict in Syria. In-patient management is necessary in many situations; however, home-based clinical management is increasingly adopted to decrease costs and improve patient experience. Home-based care has enabled some children to receive IVAB safely in their home by trained and experienced nurses and, in some instances by a parent/carer, with as little disruption to their family lives and education as possible (Jackson et al., 2022). These services have many potential benefits, including reduced hospital-acquired infections, increasing bed availability, as well as patient and family satisfaction (Bryant and Katz, 2018; Shepperd et al., 2016).

Although a home service is not suitable for all children receiving IVAB, the outreach team have discussed with the family Naajy's suitability to receive home treatment and to provide a more comfortable experience for patient and family. A training session for parents on the use of equipment and information about medicines and their side effects, as well as caring for the IV lines at home, will have to be provided before discharge (Bryant and Katz, 2018). The outreach team will be visiting the family daily to administer antibiotics, assess Naajy's wellbeing, offer support and advice to his family, make management plans and identify potential issues. It is essential that nursing staff have up to date contact details of the parents before Naajy is sent home. His parents will receive detailed written and verbal information in Arabic and the telephone number to use in case of any concerns.

Language is key to communication, as it helps the speaker and listener to understand each other's needs. The importance of being able to communicate with patients and families is paramount. Nurses are responsible for providing patient-centred care to their patients regardless of their personal characteristics including language skills (Nursing and Midwifery Council, 2018). Naajy and his family have limited English proficiency. Furthermore, Naajy and his family are learning to communicate using Makaton. This is a recognised communication system for people with learning disabilities, employed by more than 100,000 children and adults (Makaton, 2022). Considering Naajy's family's communication needs before care interventions is therefore essential, to ensure that their needs are understood and met.

The National Health Service (NHS) aims to offer high quality, patient-centred care to the diverse population it serves (Department of Health, 2012). However, language barriers negatively impact the nurses' ability to effectively assess care needs, and may lead to health and social care professionals unable to provide safe and effective care (Ali and Watson, 2018). In responding to the needs of every patient they care for; nurses cannot learn every language. However, an understanding of language barriers and their impact can help to overcome challenges to the provision of effective care (Ali and Watson, 2018). Nurses should be encouraged to be proactive and involved in policy making, providing feedback on language services within their organisations and wider health care systems.

Naajy's family uses a friend as an interpreter on a regular basis as they feel more comfortable with someone who has a better understanding of their needs. The use of untrained interpreters can be very effective, although also presents ethical and practical challenges. These relate to issues of confidentiality and also limited understanding of medical terminology and problems providing explanations to the patient. Restricting the use of medical information, may prevent opportunities for interventions and support to the family (Lucas, 2015; Dorner, Orellana-Faulstich, and Jiménez, 2010). Health professionals should balance the need for confidentiality with competent interpreting to support best care. Therefore, professional interpreting services are preferable, particularly regarding medical intervention, to help overcome language barriers which enable Naajy's family to have a better understanding about service provision and accessibility (Turnbull et al., 2019).

National and international organisations have been advocating for children's best interests for decades, notably so that their voices are heard (United Nations General Assembly, 1989; Department of Health and Children, 2000; European Association for Children in Hospital, 2002; Council of Europe, 2011). However, children's views are often obtained through proxy data by parents and may not be representative of an issue that is important to them (Dickinson, Wrapson, and Water, 2014). To achieve child participation in health and social care provision and decision-making, it is necessary to develop appropriate ways of including children and alternative methods of data collection. Studies show that children can share their views, despite concerns that they may be unreliable informants (Coyne, 2006; Coad and Coad, 2008). There are many examples in the literature, not only involving parents, but also children in the planning of new healthcare services as well as design of clinical and care-giving spaces (Coyne, 2006; Cook and Hess, 2007; Coad and Coad, 2008; Carter and Ford, 2013; Water et al., 2017).

Naajy communicates, through Makaton, that hospital environments provoke emotions such as fear, anxiety and sadness. In common with many studies, children of all ages experience similar emotions when hospitalised which adversely impacts on their physical and psychosocial wellbeing (Carney et al., 2003; Coyne, 2006; Fletcher et al., 2011; Forsner et al., 2009; Salmela et al., 2009; Wilson et al., 2010; Norton-Westwood, 2012). Art-based methods such as 'draw and tell' (in which participants are encouraged to draw and then explain their drawings) and letter writing have been found to be a valuable way to obtain children's views (Cook and Hess, 2007; Carter and Ford, 2013; Water et al., 2017). Communication can be challenging for many children with learning challenges, particularly concerning auditory and visual processing, memory and retrieval of concepts. Therefore art-based methods can be adapted for Naajy and other individuals with learning disabilities, or communication difficulties, so they can make themselves understood and the quality of care they receive is consequently increased (Neilson, 2019).

Reflection Points for Nursing Practice

- Measuring patient satisfaction is essential to improving person-centred care.
- Involvement of patients and carers in the improvement of services offers opportunities to discover what really makes a difference to their experience and provide a better understanding of their needs and priorities.
- To meet the needs of every patient they care for, nurses need to understand language barriers and their impact, as this can help to overcome challenges to effective care.
- Art-based methods can be a valuable way to obtain children's views and adaptation should be made to include the views of children with learning disabilities and/or communication difficulties.

Education

To demonstrate how Naajy and his family might become part of a PPI group and contribute to the nursing curriculum, the following evidence-based example is provided, drawing on the authors' experiences. Naajy and his family are approached for their lived experience of disability, migration, and palliative care. As touched upon in the evidence for practice chapter, this involves 'expert by experience', which draws on the life experiences of patients and their significant others to inform care. This complements more traditional expert knowledge, such as from nurses and doctors, essentially to ensure that the care provided is meaningful to the recipient (Honey et al., 2020). The family expressed a desire to share their experiences so that their knowledge can help inform and aid other refugee families. Despite encountering some poor care practices previously, they have also experienced good examples of care, which they feel could be replicated. Naajy likes the nurses who have cared for him so far and shares a desire to 'help the nurses to learn'. To commence this process, the Chairperson of the University PPI group, approached the family and explained carefully what becoming part of the PPI group would involve. She made sure the family understood the time commitments and financial acknowledgement for participating. This is important for the purposes of informed consent and agreeing to be participants. Ensuring financial recognition for PPI members' time is also important, as it highlights their valuable contributions and helps facilitate trusting and more equal partnerships (Knowles et al., 2021). The PPI Chairperson also offered a realistic perspective that the family could engage as little or as much as they wished, and not feel pressured nor overwhelmed. The family was also reassured that Naajy's medical needs, alongside the health and wellbeing of the family, should always be the priority.

When discussing the involvement Naajy and his family might have within a university nurse education programme, many considerations were needed. It was recognised that a disabled child and his carer (mother) would need to come as a pair to help Naajy feel comfortable. Farah would act as Naajy's advocate, particularly when he might struggle to understand or be understood by others. For Naajy's family, their additional language needs also meant they would require support from an interpreter. The family were already working closely with a refugee community worker, who agreed to be involved in terms of acting as an interpreter, within nursing educational activities.

Our experience has taught us that PPI should come from a place of comfort and knowledge. A recent report by Health Education England (2019) alludes to this approach, suggesting that PPI works best when mutual benefits, respect and relationships are developed. Naajy and his family were thus encouraged to speak about areas of care they felt comfortable to explore, so that their unique expertise could be valued without adding additional burdens to the family. Boundaries on what might be discussed and how this might proceed were crucial to prepare the family as well as ensure the teaching sessions were successful. By listening to the family, two separate sessions were required with the students. This was deemed most beneficial, because both the carer and child perspectives could be given equal time and value.

The first educational session for the university nurse education programme, was conducted with Farah, Naajy's mother, and the support worker. The session followed a predetermined and jointly created list of questions and topics of potential interest to the students and relating to Farah's expertise. The lecturer or support worker was able to gently prompt and question Farah about her experiences as a carer. By having a session dedicated to carer experience, Farah had longer to speak and share her own expertise first. She was able to give details of the family's history and Naajy's diagnosis for context too. Farah was also able to discuss aspects she may not have wished to share with her son present, while allowing time and attention dedicated to the students, rather than having to care, or consider her son's needs. Given that Gumm et al. (2017) found many parents and carers felt a lack of recognition of parental knowledge and experience was detrimental to their care, it was also important to honour the expertise of parents in caring for their child and to role model a family centred approach. Moreover, the refugee support worker was able to offer additional insights into the experience of refugees and their unique health care needs, building student understanding of the specific complexity of needs surrounding migration trauma, access barriers, community hostility and aspects which may optimise future care.

The second session was created to enable Naajy to interact with the student nurses directly. Naajy loves learning Makaton and anything musical. It was decided with his family, that he might teach the student nurses Makaton signs and share with them some of his favourite music accompanied with the signs. This session was also chosen to enable further learning about communication aids within learning disability nursing. Gumm et al. (2017) explore the importance of learning the signs for 'yes' and 'no' when caring for disabled children, as they explain a lot of communication can happen with just this knowledge. Further, Vinales (2013) claims that Makaton training can be invaluable for effective communication to optimise patient care.

Many factors were considered to enable this session to take place. Farah told us that Naajy would struggle to be the centre of attention in a classroom setting with lots of students. The session was therefore conducted online with a reduced number of particularly interested students, who were willing to engage with the activities. A list of common Makaton signs that might be used in a hospital setting were chosen, with students asking Naajy and his mother to show them how to sign the symbols they had in front of them and then practising them together. These were interspersed with fun signs of Naajy's choosing to help him feel more at ease such as a giraffe and other animals. The session ended with singing Naajy's favourite songs following a video demonstration. The family asked if we could also include a Syrian lullaby to share some of the family's rich cultural heritage.

In addition to integrating patient and family views into the education highlighted, when considering education and PPI, the student nurse perspective is also vital to understanding effectiveness and improving approaches. Hence in the following section, student nurses reflect on their experiences of PPI involvement with their education. One student and co-author, Beth, reflects:

> Patient and public involvement, from a student nurse's perspective, teaches you things that a textbook can't, the humanity in nursing and the nuances of each individual. People can have the same diagnosis but very different presentations and needs that can only be learnt from them and those closest to them – 'the experts by experience'.

Many benefits for patients are suggested by Health Education England (2018), including nurses working more in partnership with patients, lessening reliance on a hierarchy of clinical expertise, while developing abilities to listen and respect the views provided by the patients. Health Education England (2018) also emphasise the importance of being person-centred with the patient as an active partner, meaning that the views of patients, as well as their significant others, are pivotal to shape care that is meaningful to both parties.

It is argued that the PPI approach also challenge stereotypes, allowing for open discussions and understanding around the world the patient inhabits, to aid student nurses to see the person holistically (Health Education England, 2018). This was evident within the Makaton session with Naajy, which was designed with his expertise taking centre stage. This built on Naajy's strengths to teach the students a skill that otherwise, they may not have encountered. According to a study by Vinales (2013), 85% of students in such Makaton sessions develop ways to interact with others and, likewise, the enthusiastic and interactive session aided learning through students gaining confidence with approaching people who communicate non-verbally. The students also reported that such learning facilitates overcoming barriers in care, particularly when issues around communication could negatively impact the patient and their family. For example, when there was non-engagement from clinicians and inaccessibility to service provision (Vinales, 2013). Predominantly, research has found positive responses from students who have had PPI integrated into their nursing programmes. 84% of students asked found the PPI member helpful and 77% found the sessions assisted their learning (Kuti and Houghton, 2019). However, reviews investigating the impact of PPI on nurse education acknowledge that there is limited research available. Therefore, more is needed to understand the benefits of this resource and to explore how it can be used to its full potential (Suikkala et al., 2018).

There is evidence that embedding PPI as part of the education programme delivery enriches student open-mindedness, curiosity and critical thinking about patient needs (Horgan et al., 2021). The long-term consistency of PPI involvement enables students to familiarise themselves with patients, enrich ways to build therapeutic relationships alongside the promotion of curiosity about holistic needs (Ferri et al., 2019). From a student perspective, there is always more to learn although it is not always possible to be taught by a PPI member associated with every disease/disability. For example employing a PPI member to share experiences of more common conditions they may encounter in practice, such as chronic obstructive pulmonary disease, to build understanding from a patient perspective. Nevertheless, the benefit of meeting PPI members with rare illnesses cannot be denied. They are the true experts, while the illnesses explored might be unfamiliar to many professionals, denoting that otherwise, knowledge of such conditions might be unattainable. This is while Atkinson and Williams (2011) suggest that, for a number of patients, student engagement is often a cherished experience.

In conclusion, many benefits exist of the long-term nature of PPI relationships and involvement in nursing programmes, which is supported by the literature. Fukuo et al. (2019) suggest that PPI needs to be part of a long-term sustained commitment for better cultural understanding and to extend areas of involvement to those with expertise by experience. Continued shared dialogue has enabled PPI members to influence the curriculum in many ways including teaching and assessing students. The leadership and strategic understanding and commitment to PPI, as seen with involving Naajy and his family to teach nursing students, can also be crucial for nurse educator's abilities to support, develop and embed PPI throughout the nursing programme (Health Education England, 2019).

Reflection Points for Education

- Comfort and knowledge – listen to what the PPI member wants to help with and ascertain what their area of expertise is.
- Make any involvement bespoke to improve meeting individual needs and preferences, within a collaborative approach.
- Ensure clear and transparent explanations for what might be involved when trying to enhance the curriculum. Preparation and frequent communication are therefore key to successful educational activities.
- A varied PPI team helps to provide diverse expertise and experience which is important for all branches of nursing. However, it is not possible to provide examples of every condition, but variety of experience can help to enhance the specific and general aspects of care informed by the patient's expertise.
- Commitment to PPI by both the nurse education team and PPI members is crucial in terms of time, financial acknowledgement for contributions, but also mutual respect and relationship building.

Research

Patient and public involvement and our understanding of the approach has advanced in recent years, with an appreciation that expertise can come from lived experiences (Grant and Ramcharan, 2010). Consequently, PPI philosophy suggests that research participants also have unique perspectives and insights to share rather than seen simply as objects of enquiry (Shaw, Brady, and Davey, 2011; Serrant, 2020). Such acknowledgement has promoted many research funding organisations and ethical approval bodies to routinely ask for PPI within funding and research ethics applications. However, there is a tendency to offer tokenistic, limited or unauthentic approaches to PPI, simply to satisfy such requirements (Knowles et al., 2021). Subsequently, evidence-based approaches are needed to ensure PPI is meaningful, with active participation and empowerment, so to influence and affect positive change within health and social care research (National Institute for Health Research, 2015; Serrant, 2020).

The Ladder of Engagement offers a framework for understanding levels of PPI involvement which is adapted from Arnstein's work in 1969. The framework provides useful guidance for ascertaining the level of PPI within a research project (NHS England, 2015). At the bottom of the ladder is the *informing stage*. While the stage is crucial, it is perhaps the most simplistic and involves giving information about the research project to PPI members, which may help to understand more about the research project. Thereafter, and perhaps used sequentially is the *consulting stage*. Within consultation PPI members may be asked for feedback on research decisions or analysis, examples include surveys, panels or focus groups to ascertain viewpoints. While this stage is often the most utilised, it is also the most contested, for although consultation may be sought, PPI views may or may not influence the final outcomes.

On the third rung of the ladder is the *involving stage* and relates to direct involvement with communities/PPI members to ensure concerns are understood and more fully considered. Despite PPI perhaps influencing aspects of the research within this stage, researchers still make the final decisions. Next comes the *collaboration stage* in which partnership in each aspect of decision making is advocated, including elements of co-design. Lastly, the top of the ladder signifies the *devolving stage* in which decision-making is placed back with the community. Here PPI members work together with researchers to share, negotiate and collaborate in as many aspects of the study as possible (Auckland, 2010; Hogg, 2015). Within this gold standard stage, PPI are considered partners within design, delivery, and research evaluation, with equal influence and examples of co-production (NHS England, 2015). Co-production aims to move beyond academic 'ivory towers', involving dynamic partnerships with people directly impacted by the subject under investigation, to improve the relevance, sensitivity, and impact of research (Greenhalgh et al., 2016; Redman et al., 2021).

Families, such as Naajy's, are often seen as 'hard to reach' within research literature, subsequently their voices may be missing from crucial discourses about their healthcare needs (Hussain, Koffman, and Bajwah, 2021). It is important to acknowledge that viewing ethnically diverse communities as 'hard to reach', can encourage a view that they are somehow 'deficient, lacking or inferior, and in need of services which will enrich their behaviour' (Hussain, Koffman, and Bajwah, 2021, p. 811). Rather, we ascertain that families, like Naajy's, are not 'hard to reach' but that the current dominant practices of engagement with patients and the public have not been fully considered to ensure accessibility for all. Therefore, it is our PPI engagement practices which need to be readdressed and assessed for their inclusivity. This element of the chapter thus hopes to provide guidance as to how PPI within research might offer approaches to reach all communities, and foster community engagement which aims to equalise some of the power imbalances seen within research.

Barriers, when exploring PPI within research, include the investment and additional time to facilitate authentic methods of engagement. It can be difficult to find, create, fund, and sustain PPI groups particularly for early career researchers or those with limited or no research budgets. Hence, it is advocated that researchers explore the advisory groups which may already exist for their area of research. When researching complex issues which interconnect for families such as Naajy's, including migration, child health and palliative care, it may be advisable to seek different groups to gain differing expertise in each area. One advantage of utilising pre-existing advisory groups is that the researcher will likely become an agenda item with oversight for their interactions, time involvement and requests being led by PPI chairs. An additional benefit is recognised within the corresponding readdressing of typical authoritative researcher hierarchy (National Institute for Health Research, 2015; Auckland, 2010; Shaw, Brady, and Davey, 2011), as the researcher is not in control but rather becomes part of a larger network, able to draw on specific PPI expertise (Brett et al., 2014).

A further suggestion to increase authentic PPI is a commitment to long-term involvement and working closely with community organisations in an area of interest. By getting to know PPI members, researchers may improve abilities to develop a 'space to talk and change'. These elements are considered vital for honest feedback, to sit with and respond to tensions, and enhancing shared dialogue with PPI members (Knowles et al., 2021). For many members of ethnically diverse communities, particularly those who may feel marginalised such as Naajy's family, the building of trusting relationships over time is crucial to having open conversations. PPI members need to feel able to give feedback and voice their honest opinions, particularly if they disagree with the researcher. These aspects of PPI relationships are crucial if researchers want to ratify, question, challenge or truly contextualise their research findings (Serrant-Green, 2011).

A further consideration when working in refugee health and social care research is that of accessibility and inclusivity. How do we involve refugee families, if their first language is not English, while they have experienced migration trauma, and community hostility? This suggests that the families will be reticent to talk to researchers, while Ziersch et al. (2019) state that a central aspect of research with refugee communities is that of close community collaboration to ensure authenticity. Working closely with communities, charities, and refugee organisations is advised so that professional interpreters and trusted translators can be used, and researchers may enhance their understanding of the constraints and needs that families may have.

A further recommendation is the use of a cultural humility stance within research. Cultural humility moves away from traditional cultural competence frameworks. Cultural competence while encouraging learning, increased awareness and cultural knowledge (McKenzie, 2008), has been criticised for not fully acknowledging the complexities of culture. The idea that one can complete a cultural skill set is overly simplistic and has the potential for an overestimation of personal competence levels, which may encourage arrogance, precipitate misunderstandings and lead to ethnic reductionism and stereotyping (Culley, 2014). Rather, cultural humility offers an approach in which self-reflection, introspection and co-learning are central principles (Tervalon and Murray-Garcia, 1998). When using this stance or philosophy researchers are encouraged to be humble and offer their incompetence - 'I do not know about this', using such openness as an invitation for participants to educate them – 'please tell me more' (Yeager and Bauer-Wu, 2013). For example, within interactions with Naaji's family a researcher may acknowledge their own unfamiliarity of the family's Muslim faith and thereby may ask the family to further explain the faith to aid the researcher's understanding. The approach may seem simple, but to offer such humility, shows respect to the family, and the value of their expertise. Ziersch et al. (2019) detail the importance of PPI approaches which allow refugee participants to 'lead' the direction of their responses rather than following a pre-determined schedule. Such approaches are thought to empower PPI members, by providing more control over the topics covered in conversations, thus, enabling PPI members to offer broader contexts not conceived by the researcher.

Finally, a consideration of creative approaches is advocated to provide additional opportunities for enhanced expression. When English is a second language, aspects such as photography, art or poetry may be particularly beneficial with helping PPI members or research participants to articulate their thoughts, feelings, and experiences more clearly (Liamputtong et al., 2008). The use of creative methods which are chosen by the PPI member, or research participant, may also help to limit concerns that researchers often focus on an elite view which favours those eloquent with speaking the English language (Tuffour, 2017). Refugee families may prefer to discuss a family photograph or artefact of personal significance, or may feel better able to give their opinions and experiences when discussing their or another's poetry or artwork. Through using such additional approaches with PPI/research interactions, families may feel more at ease, facilitating the building of rapport and relationships with the families.

When considering the involvement of children themselves in research activities, efforts should be made to include a range of ages, populations, and contexts, to broaden and enhance research findings. Utilising small group activities, arts-based approaches and community participation can help with recruitment and retainment of children and young people (Rouncefield-Swales et al., 2021). A cultural humility approach can be similarly beneficial by offering non-hierarchical perspectives that support and value all elements of participation. Flexibility in terms of levels of involvement with children and young people is crucial to ensuring choice, meeting of individual preferences and respect for the level of time, skill, or ability available (Rouncefield-Swales et al., 2021).

Researchers also need to consider the benefits to children and young people with being involved in research. Participation in research can offer valuable ways of contributing to health care improvements, having their voices heard and give opportunities for wider research impact (Rouncefield-Swales et al., 2021). However, many researchers may be concerned about the potential for harm to children and young people from research involvement. Graham et al. (2013) state that concerns around protecting children should not be used as a research inclusion or exclusion criteria. Instead, it should serve as a prompt to ensuring children and young people's involvement is contextual, consent driven and age appropriate. Thus, the key principles of safety, inclusion and empowerment are vital when considering the ethical involvement of children and young people in research activities (Graham et al., 2013).

Reflection Points for Research

- The use of pre-existing advisory groups may offer pragmatic but also power equalising benefits for researchers.
- Community, charity, and refugee organisations offer valuable sources of expertise and may help to increase validity, sensitivity, and appropriateness to interactions with refugee families.
- A cultural humility approach is valuable in PPI/research interactions and may help to value, respect and encourage two-way educational approaches with families.
- Creative approaches may also help refugee families to voice their opinions, give more detail and enhance rapport and relationship building.
- Children and young people have important perspectives to enhance health care research. Ways to involve them in research which consider their abilities, preferences, and context are thus needed.

Conclusion

This chapter outlined how student and registered nurses can work in partnership with patients, family members, informal caregivers, and members of PPI groups upholding the principle 'nothing about us without us'. An anonymised scenario, relating to Naajy and his family, guided the application of the PPI pillar to nursing practice, education, and research. Involvement of patients and carers in the improvement of services offers opportunities to discover what really makes differences to their experiences and provide better understanding of their needs and priorities. Evaluating patient satisfaction is essential to improving patient-centred care. Moreover, to meet the needs of every patient they care for, nurses need to understand language barriers and their impact, as this can help to overcome challenges to provide effective care. Art-based methods can be a valuable way to obtain children's views, and adaptation should be made to include the views of children with learning disabilities and/or communication difficulties within their care.

Commitment to PPI by both nurse education teams and PPI members is crucial in terms of time, financial acknowledgement for contributions, but also mutual respect and relationship building. A varied PPI team helps to provide diverse expertise and experience, important for all branches of nursing, by helping to enhance understanding specific and general aspects of care. A collaborative approach is key to ensure bespoke involvement to meet individuals' needs and preferences, as well as clear and transparent communication and guidelines with the involvement of curriculum enhancement.

Finally, the use of pre-existing advisory groups may offer pragmatic but also power equalising benefits for researchers. Community, charity, and refugee organisations offer valuable sources of expertise and may help to increase authenticity, sensitivity, and appropriateness to interactions with refugee families. A Cultural Humility approach is valuable in PPI/research interactions and may help to value, respect, and encourage reciprocal educational approaches with families. Creative approaches may also help refugee families to voice their opinions, provide more detail, enhance rapport as well as building relationships. Children and young people have important perspectives to enhance health care research, highlighting that when involving children in research, their abilities, preferences, and contexts – and those of their families – remain central to care planning and decision-making.

Takeaways for Student Nurses, Educators, and Practitioners

- Involvement of PPI members can improve and encourage individualised, person-centred care and enhance the nursing evidence base.
- Always listen to and work towards activities which suit the PPI members area of expertise –PPI comes best from a place of 'comfort and knowledge'.
- A collaborative ethos is essential for authentic PPI and the building of mutual respect. Preparation, transparency of expectations and frequent communication can be the key.
- Meaningful dialogue with PPI members includes a commitment to building safe, trusted relationships, which offer the space to 'talk, challenge, and change'.
- Creative arts-based methods can be valuable, particularly when seeking children/young people's views or those whose first language is not English.
- The involvement of community, charitable organisations and existing PPI groups may help to enhance sensitivity and understanding of patient perspectives within nurse education, practice, and research.

Media Resources about Patient and Public Involvement

- TED talk, 'Cultural Humility' by Juliana Mosley, PhD (available at: www.you tube.com/watch?v=Ww_ml21L7Ns).
- BBC Radio podcast, 'Ouch! . . . The cabin fever podcast' by Beth Rose, Emma Tracey, Keiligh Baker, and Kate Monaghan (available at: Access All: Disability News and Mental Health – Welcome to The Cabin Fever Podcast – BBC Sounds).
- Health Talk offer patient perspectives and additional insights into care (available at: www.healthtalk.org).
- TED talk, 'The Danger of a Single Story' by Chimamanda Ngozi Adichie, novelist (available at: www.ted.com/talks/chimamanda_adichie_the_danger_of_a_ single_story?language=en).

References

Adstamongkonkul, D. and Hess, D. (2017) 'Ischemic Conditioning and neonatal hypoxic ischemic encephalopathy: a literature review', *Conditioning Medicine*, 1(1), pp. 9–16.

Ali, P. and Watson, R. (2018) 'Language barriers and their impact on provision of care to patients with limited English proficiency: Nurses' perspectives', *Journal of Clinical Nursing*, 27(5–6), pp. 1–9.

Arnstein, S.R. (1969) 'A ladder of citizen participation', *Journal of American Planning Association*, 35(4), pp. 216–224.

Atkinson, S. and Williams, P. (2011) 'The involvement of service users in nursing students' education', *Learning Disability Practice*, 14(3), pp. 18–21.

Auckland, S. (2010) *BRC Guidance: Involving users in research*. Available at: www.acprc.org.uk/ Data/Resource_Downloads/a_how_to_guide_for_researchers.pdf (Accessed: 12 December 2022).

Batalden, P. and Davidoff, F. (2007) 'What is "quality improvement" and how can it transform healthcare?', *Quality and Safety in Health Care*, 16(1), pp. 2–3.

Brett, J. Staniszewska, S. Mockford, C. Herron-Marx, S. Hughes, J. Tysall, C.A. (2014) 'A Systematic Review of the Impact of Patient and Public Involvement on Service Users, Researchers and Communities', *Patient*, 7, pp. 387–395.

Bryant, P. and Katz, N. (2018) 'Inpatient versus parenteral antibiotic therapy at home for acute infections in children: a systematic review', *The lancet Infectious Diseases*, 18(2), pp. 1–10.

Carney, T., Murphy, S., McClure, J., Bishop, E., Kerr, C., Parker, J., Scott, F., Shields, C. and Wilson, L. (2003) 'Children's views of hospitalisation: An exploratory study of data collection', *Journal of Child Health Care*, 7(1), pp. 27–40.

Carter, B., and Ford, K. (2013) 'Researching children's health experiences: The place for participatory, child centred, arts-based approaches', *Research in Nursing and Health*, 36(1), 95–107.

Charlton, J.I. (2000) *Nothing about us without us: Disability oppression and empowerment*. Berkeley, CA: University of California Press.

Coad, J. and Coad, N. (2008) 'Children and young people's preference of thematic design and colour for their hospital environment', *Journal of Child Health Care*, 12, pp. 33–48.

Cook, T. and Hess, E. (2007) 'What the camera sees and from whose perspective Fun methodologies for engaging children in enlightening adults', *Childhood*, 14(1), pp. 29–45.

Council of Europe. (2011) *Guidelines on child-friendly health care*. Available at: 168046ccef (coe. int) (Accessed: 10 January 2023).

Coyne, I. (2006) 'Children's experiences of hospitalization', *Journal of Child Health Care*, 10(4), pp. 326–336.

Culley, L. (2014) 'Editorial: Nursing and super-diversity', *Journal of Research in Nursing*, 19(6), pp. 453–455.

Department of Health. (2012) 'Compassion in practice. Nursing, midwifery and care staff. Our vision and strategy'. Available at: www.england.nhs.uk/wp-content/uploads/2012/12/compas sion-in-practice.pdf (Accessed: 13 January 2023).

Department of Health and Children. (2000) *National Children's Strategy: Our Children – Their Lives*. Dublin: The Stationery Office.

Department of Health and Social Care. (2012) 'The NHS Constitution for England'. Available at: www.gov.uk/government/publications/the-nhs-constitution-for-england/the-nhs-constitution-for-england (Accessed: 20 January 2023).

Dickinson, A., Wrapson, W. and Water, T. (2014) 'Children's voices in public hospital health-care delivery: Intention as opposed to practice', *The New Zealand Medical Journal*, 127(1405), pp. 24–31.

Dorner, L., Orellana-Faulstich, M. and Jiménez, R. (2010) 'It's one of those things that you do to help the family': language brokering and the development of immigrant adolescents, *Journal of Adolescent Research*, 23(5), pp. 515–543.

Entwistle, V., Renfrew, M., Forrester, J. and Lamont, T. (1998) 'Lay perspectives: advantages for health research', *BMJ*, 316(7129), pp. 463–466.

European Association for Children in Hospital. (2002) *The EACH Charter for Children in Hospital and Annotations*. Dublin: Children in Hospital Ireland.

Ferri, P., Rovesti, S., Padula, M.S., D'Amico, R. and Di Lorenzo, R. (2019) 'Effect of expert-patient teaching on empathy in nursing students: a randomized controlled trial', *Psychology Research and Behavior Management*, 12, pp. 457–467.

Fletcher, T., Glasper, A., Prudhoe, G., Battrick, C., Coles, L., Weaver, K. and Ireland, L. (2011) 'Building on the future: Children's views on nurses and hospital care', *British Journal of Nursing*, 20(1), pp. 39–45.

Forsner, M., Jansson, L. and Soderberg, A. (2009) 'Afraid of medical care: School-aged children's narratives about medical fear', *Journal of Pediatric Nursing*, 24(6), pp. 519–528.

Fukuo, J.F., Maroney, M.M. and Corrigan, P. (2019) 'Pilot of a consumer based anti-stigma mentorship program for nursing students', *Journal of Public Mental Health*, 19 (1), pp. 51–61.

Graham, A., Powell, M., Taylor, N., Anderson, D., and Fitzgerald, R. (2013) 'Ethical research involving children. UNICEF Office of Research–Innocenti. Available at: http://childethics.com/ (Accessed 26 April 2023).

Grant, G. and Ramcharan, P. (2010) 'User Involvement in Research', in K. Gerrish and K. Lacey (Eds) *The Research Process in Nursing*, 6th edition. Chichester: Blackwell Publishing, pp. 36–49.

Greco, P., Nencini, G., Piva, I., Scioscia, M., Volta, C.A., Spadaro, S., Neri, M., Bonaccorsi, G., Greco, F., Cocco, I., Sorrentino, F., D'Antonio, F., and Nappi, L. (2020) 'Pathophysiology of hypoxic-ischemic encephalopathy: a review of the past and a view on the future', *Acta Neuro-logica Belgica*, 120, pp. 277–288.

Greenhalgh, T. Jackson, C Shaw, S. and Janamian, T. (2016) 'Achieving research impact through co-creation in community-based health services: literature review and case study', *The Millbank Quarterly*, 94(2), pp. 392–429.

Gumm, R. Thomas, E. Llyod, C. Hambly, H. Tomlinson, R. Logan, S. and Morris, C. (2017) 'Improving communication between staff and disabled children in hospital wards: testing the feasibility of a training intervention developed through intervention mapping', *BMJ Paediatrics Open*, 1(1), pp. 1–7.

Health Education England. (2019) 'Pathways to embed patient and public involvement in healthcare scientist training programmes'. Available at: https://nshcs.hee.nhs.uk/wp-content/up loads/2019/08/hcs-pathways-and-ppi-report.pdf (Accessed: 7 February 2023)

Health Education England. (2018) 'Patient and public involvement in nurse education'. Available at: www.hee.nhs.uk/our-work/patient-public-involvement-nurse-education (Accessed: 5 February 2023)

Hogg, R. (2015) 'A guide to research for nurses and midwives NHS GGC'. Available at: www. nhsggc.org.uk/media/234385/beginnersguidetoresearchfinal.pdf (Accessed: 12 December 2022)

Honey, Boydell, K. M., Coniglio, F., Do, T. T., Dunn, L., Gill, K., Glover, H., Hines, M., Scanlan, J. N., and Tooth, B. (2020) 'Lived experience research as a resource for recovery: a mixed methods study', *BMC Psychiatry*, 20(1). Available at: https://bmcpsychiatry.biomedcentral.com/articles/10.1186/s12888-020-02861-0 (Accessed: 3 January 2023).

Horgan, A., Donovan, M.O., Doody, R., Savage, E., Dorrity, C., O'Sullivan, H., Goodwin, J., Greaney, S., Biering, P., Bjornsson, E. and Bocking, J. (2021) 'Improving service user involvement in mental health nursing education: Suggestions from those with lived experience', *Issues in Mental Health Nursing*, 42(2), pp. 119–127.

Hussain, J. A. Koffman, J. and Bajwah, S. (2021) 'Racism and palliative care', *Palliative Medicine*, 35(5), pp. 810–813.

Institute of Medicine. (2001) *Crossing the Quality Chasm: A New Health System for the 21st Century*. Washington, DC: National Academy Press. Available at: www.ncbi.nlm.nih.gov/books/NBK222274/?report=reader (Accessed: 12 January 2023).

INVOLVE (2013) 'Values, principles and standards for public involvement in research'. Available at: INVOLVE-Principles-and-standards-for-public-involvement-1-November-2013.pdf (Accessed: 1 February 2023).

Jackson, T., Napper, R., Haesler, B., Pizer, B., Bate, J., Grundy, R., Samarasinghe, S., Anfelini, P., Ball-Gamble, A., Phillips, B. and Morgan, J. (2022) 'Can I go home now? The safety and efficacy of a new UK paediatric febrile neutropenia protocol for risk-stratified early discharge on oral antibiotics', *Archives of Disease in Childhood*, in press.

Jensen, J., Allen, L., Blasko., R. and Nagy, P. (2016) 'Using Quality Improvement methods to Improve Patient Experience', *Journal of the American College of Radiology*, 13(12), pp. 1550–1554.

Knowles, S.E., Allen, D., Donnelly, A., Flynn, J., Gallacher, K., Lewis, A., McCorkle, G., Mistry, M., Walkington, P. and Drinkwater, J. (2021) 'More than a method: trusting relationships, productive tensions, and two-way learning as mechanisms of authentic co-production', *Research Involvement and Engagement*, 7(1), pp. 1–14.

Kuti, B., and Houghton, T. (2019) 'Service user involvement in teaching and learning: student nurse perspectives', *Journal of Research in Nursing*, 24(3–4), pp. 183–194.

Liamputtong, P. Rumbold, J. Aldridge, D. Alexander, L. Allen, J. and Bagley, C. (2008) *Knowing Differently: Arts-Based and Collaborative Research Methods*. New York: Nova Science Publishers.

Lucas, S. (2015) 'Child interpreting in social work: competence versus legitimacy', *Transnational Social Review*, 5(2), pp. 145–160.

Makaton. (2022) Available at: Home (makaton.org) (Accessed: 1 February 2023).

McKenzie, K. (2008) 'A historical perspective of cultural competence', *Ethnicity and Inequalities in Health and Social Care*, 1 (1), pp. 5–8.

Mockford, C., Staniszewska, S., Griffiths, F. and Herron-Marx, S. (2012) 'The impact of patient and public involvement on the UK NHS health care: a systematic review', *International Journal for Quality in Health Care*, 24(1), pp. 28–38.

National Institute for Health Research (2015) 'Young person's advisory group'. Available at: www.nihr.ac.uk/blog/young-people-are-the-future/20148 (Accessed: 1st February 2023).

Neilson, S. (2019) 'Using draw-and-tell methods to inform clinical nursing assessments with children aged 6–12 years', *Evidence Based Nursing*, 22(4), p. 1.

NHS England. (2015) 'Planning for participation'. Available at: www.england.nhs.uk/wp-content/uploads/2014/03/bs-guide-plann-part1.pdf (Accessed: 1 February 2023).

Norton-Westwood, D. (2012) 'The health-care environment through the eyes of a child – does it soothe or provoke anxiety?', *International Journal of Nursing Practice*, 18, pp. 7–11.

Nursing and Midwifery Council. (2018) 'The Code. Professional standards of practice and behaviour for nurses and midwives'. Available at: www.nmc.org.uk/standards/code/ (Accessed: 9 January 2023).

Redman, S. Greenhalgh, T. Adedokun, L. Straniszewska, S. and Denegri, S. (2021) 'Co-production of knowledge: the future', *BMJ*, 372, pp. 1–2.

Rouncefield-Swales, A., Harris, J., Carter, B., Bray, L., Bewley, T. and Martin, R. (2021) 'Children and young people's contributions to public involvement and engagement activities in health-related research; A scoping review', *PLoS One*, 16(6), pp. 1–25.

Salmela, M., Salanterä, S. and Aronen, E. (2009) Child-reported hospital fears in 4 to 6-year-old children', *Pediatric Nursing*, 35(5), pp. 269–276.

Serrant, L. (2020) 'Silenced Knowing: An intersectional framework for exploring black women's health and diasporic identities', *Frontiers in Sociology*, 5(1), pp. 1–9.

Serrant-Green, L. (2011) 'The sound of 'silence': A framework for researching sensitive issues or marginalised perspectives in health', *Journal of Research in Nursing*, 16(4), pp. 347–360.

Shaw, C. Brady, L. and Davey, C. (2011) 'Guidelines for research with children and young people'. Available at: https://info.lse.ac.uk/staff/divisions/research-and-innovation/research/Assets/Documents/PDF/NCB-guidelinesCYP-2011.pdf (Accessed: 12 December 2022).

Shepperd, S., Iliffe, S., Doll, H., Clarke, M., Kalra, L., Wilson, A. and Gonçalves-Bradley, D. (2016) 'Admission avoidance hospital at home', *Cochrane Database of Systematic Reviews*, 8(4), pp. 1–63.

Smith, I., Hicks, C. and McGovern, T. (2020) 'Adapting Lean methods to facilitate stakeholder engagement and co-design in healthcare', *British Medical Journal*, 368, pp. 34–37.

Suikkala, A., Koskinen, S. and Leino-Kilpi, H. (2018). 'Patients' involvement in nursing students' clinical education: A scoping review'. *International Journal of Nursing Studies*, 84, pp. 40–51.

Tallentire, V., Harley, C. and Watson, S. (2019) 'Quality planning for impactful improvement: a mixed methods review', *BMJ Open Quality*; 8, pp. 1–6.

Tervalon, M. Murray-Garcia, J. (1998) 'Cultural humility versus cultural competence: A critical distinction in defining physician training outcomes in multicultural education', *Journal of Health Care for the Poor and Underserved*, 9(2), pp. 117–125.

Thompson, A. (2015) 'Paediatric palliative care'. Symposium: Special Needs. Paediatrics and Child Health, 2510), pp. 458–462.

Tuffour, I. (2017) 'A critical overview of interpretative phenomenological analysis: a contemporary qualitative research approach', *Journal of Healthcare Communications*, 2(4), pp. 52–57.

Turnbull, J., Arenth, J., Payne, K., Lantos, J. and Fanning, J. (2019) 'When only family is available to interpret', *Pediatrics*, 143(4), pp. 1–4.

United Nations General Assembly (1989) 'Convention on the rights of the child, 20 November 1989, UN, treaty series 1577'. Available at: www.refworld.org/docid/3ae6b38f0.html (Accessed: 26 April 2023)

Vinales, J. J. (2013) 'Evaluation of Makaton in practice by children's nursing' students', *Nursing Children and Young People*, 25(3) pp. 14–17.

Water, T., Wrapson, J., Tokolahi, E., Payam, S. and Reay, S. (2017) 'Participatory art-based research with children to gain their perspectives on designing healthcare environments', *Contemporary Nurse*, 53(4), pp. 456–473.

Wilson, M., Megel, M., Enenbach, L. and Carlson, K. (2010) 'The voices of children: Stories about hospitalization, *Journal of Pediatric Health Care*, 24(2), pp. 95–102.

Wilson, P., Mathie, E., Keenan, J., McNeilly, E., Goodman, C., Howe, A., Poland, F., Staniszweska, S., Kendall, S., Munday, D. and Cowe, M. (2015) 'ReseArch with Patient and Public invOlvement: a realisT evaluation: the RAPPORT study. Health services and delivery research'. Available at: https://uhra.herts.ac.uk/handle/2299/23531 (Accessed; 26 April 2023).

Yeager, K.A. and Bauer-Wu, S. (2013) 'Cultural humility: essential foundation for clinical researchers', *Applied Nursing Research*, 26(4), pp. 251–256.

Ziersch, A., Due, C., Arthurson, K. and Loehr, N. (2019) 'Conducting Ethical Research with People from Asylum Seeker and Refugee Backgrounds', in P. Liamputtong (ed.), *Handbook of Research Methods in Health Social Sciences*. Singapore: Springer, pp. 1871–1889.

6 No Health without Mental Health Pillar

*Rachel Miller, Jemima Kempton, Hayley Rich,
Oreoluwa Onifade, Simon Privett,
Kris Deering, and Mary Mancini*

Introduction

The chapter considers wide-ranging health related factors that intersect with mental health and include the biological, psychological, and social contexts that intertwine with wellbeing and shape our lives. We introduce an anonymised scenario of 'Matthew' who is experiencing low mood and alcohol use. Following an overview of the links between mental health and physical health conditions, we then apply elements of scholarship relating to the 'no health without mental health' pillar to illuminate elements of Matthew's experience. The aim is to consider mental health related strategies to assist Matthew drawing on ideas which include recovery, holism and person-centeredness. Thereafter, a fuller account of holistic care and its importance in meeting the needs of the whole person, is provided. This is developed in the concluding section about recovery-focused approaches and coordination to ensure, whenever possible, that the patient voice, as well as personal attributes contributes to their care.

Scenario

Matthew is a forty-one-year-old male, who worked in the British Army for twenty years. He served in the infantry and was stationed in the UK, Germany, Gibraltar, and Kenya. Matthew enjoyed his time with the armed forces, stating that it helped him find structure and purpose, following a difficult upbringing. He valued the peer support and comradery the military offered him and was particularly proud to represent the Army as a rugby player. Matthew played as a prop forward and sustained many injuries over a decade, including a dislocated right shoulder. Matthew's shoulder injuries never fully healed, leaving Matthew with musculoskeletal damage to his shoulder, which resulted in a medical discharge from the Army. Since then, Matthew has struggled to maintain employment due to a decline in his physical and mental health. He is currently unemployed and receives state benefits including disability allowance.

Matthew describes the challenges of living with chronic pain. He experienced a significant dip in his mood and had become increasingly isolated and agitated, which he attributed to the breakdown of his marriage. Matthew's divorce from his wife, Steph, was acrimonious and resulted in only supervised access to his children, Marcus (aged 7) and Evie (aged 6). Matthew

DOI: 10.4324/9781003390565-6

also describes disturbed sleep, reporting sleeping only 4 hours per night. He says he drinks up to half a bottle of whiskey (20 units) to 'help' his sleep and 'take the edge off the pain'. Some evenings, Matthew will drink in the local bar where he has a few acquaintances, although these are not close, and he feels unable to speak about his difficulties.

Matthew's injury and pain is managed by a local doctor and the Pain Management Consultant at the nearby hospital, where he has been trialling different treatments with no success so far. Matthew feels constantly tired, and he has lost interest in preparing nutritious meals resulting in Matthew gaining weight. He reports struggling with his self-esteem and overall loss of identities including his relationships: as a father, within work, as a rugby player and as a person within his community. Compounded by the experience of chronic pain, Matthew reports feeling hopeless and worthless, and regularly questions what is left for him in life.

Due to the stressors that Matthew is facing, including elevated alcohol consumption, increased agitation, disturbed sleep, increased weight and reported low mood, Matthew is currently under review by his practice nurse who is dual qualified in adult and mental health nursing. He is also being monitored for potential Type 2 diabetes (nonhereditary increase in blood glucose), which was highlighted following a recent NHS Health Check. This is very worrying for Matthew, as his father died two years ago from complications related to Type 2 diabetes.

Overview of Mental Health

Experiences of mental health are personal to each of us, beginning at the microscopic level of human biology, including the close relationships within which our bodies, brains and personalities develop and moving outwards to our collective existence. This includes the socioeconomic and political contexts that shape our health and wellbeing (Maté and Maté, 2022). Globally, nearly one billion people live with a mental health condition, from depression, anxiety and substance misuse to neuro-development disorders, psychosis, and dementia. However, mental health remains one of the most neglected aspects of healthcare (World Health Organization, 2022) with global governments spending, on average, just over 2% of their health budgets on mental health (World Health Organization, 2020). Furthermore, poor mental health was estimated to cost the world economy approximately $2.5 trillion per year in poor health and reduced productivity in 2010, a cost projected to rise to $6 trillion by 2030 (Lancet Global Health, 2020).

Spending might also be a question about distribution, with a sizeable portion of budgets expended on medication overlooking the social, political, and economic determinants of mental health (Rajkumar, 2022). Moreover, centralised governments tend to work in silos, and lack partnerships with health services influencing the amount funded, while countries with high mortality rates owing to infectious diseases see mental health as less of a priority (Liu et al., 2017; Rathod et al., 2017). Cultural factors also have bearing, given the differences globally in how mental health is perceived, and the degrees associated with stigma which influence expenditure (Alloh et al., 2018). Furthermore, distribution from health budgets vary, the Organisation for Economic Co-operation and Development (2021) propose Norway and Sweden spend the most per capita on mental health care, correlated to higher taxes to fund services (Pedersen, 2019). Interestingly, funding does not necessarily correlate to patient satisfaction, and can depend on the care approaches provided (Mahomed, 2020). Hence, much complexity is at play regarding financing, and caution is required around suggestions that one, or two causal factors explain all issues relating to mental health funding.

Nevertheless, it is difficult to deny the amount of literature substantiating the vast global inequalities with access and delivery of mental health resources (Patel et al., 2018). To achieve the global objectives set out in the WHO comprehensive mental health action plan 2013–2030 (World Health Organization, 2021) and the Sustainable Development Goals (United Nations (UN), 2015), there is a need to transform our attitudes, actions, and approaches towards mental health and how we provide care for those in need (World Health Organization, 2022). This raises the question around how health and care workers, educators, researchers, and leaders can provide strategic guidance, evidence, tools, and scholarship to address the link between the mind and body. Included are considerations around the influences of relationships, social circumstances, history and culture on our health, wellbeing, and sense of self.

No Health without Mental Health Pillar Overview

It is important to recognise that our mental health is not shaped in a vacuum and is impacted by multiple systemic, cultural, relational, and political landscapes. The inescapable links between our emotions, culture, bodies, and spirits are well established. For example, research indicates:

- People with chronic physical health conditions are 2 to 3 times more likely to develop a mental health condition (Barnett et al., 2012; Naylor et al., 2012; King's Fund, 2012; National Institute of Mental Health, 2021).
- People with two or more chronic physical health conditions are up to 7 times more likely to experience depression (Ronaldson et al., 2021; National Institute of Mental Health, 2021).
- Adults with childhood trauma are more likely to use substances, experience poor physical and mental health, and die prematurely (Ashton et al., 2016a, 2016b; Bellis et al., 2019; Brown et al., 2009; Hughes et al., 2017).
- Children who encounter 4 or more adverse childhood experiences (ACES) are 4 times more likely to develop type 2 diabetes, 3 times more likely to develop respiratory conditions, and three times more likely to develop heart disease (Bellis et al., 2019).
- People with serious mental illness (SMI – for example schizophrenia, bipolar and borderline personality disorder) are more likely to die prematurely than people without such a condition (Public Health England, 2018; Schneider et al., 2019). In England for instance, people with SMI are 4.5 times more likely to die before the age of 75 (Office for Health Improvements and Disparities, 2023).
- Social isolation is associated with increased risk of mortality in countries at different economic levels (Naito et al., 2021).
- Workplace culture has been identified as a risk factor for an individual's mental health and wellbeing, with employees identifying their managers as having a bigger impact (either positively or negatively) on their mental health, than their doctors or therapists; with the same impact as the employee's spouse or partner (Workforce Institute, 2023).
- Furthermore, armed conflicts, natural disasters and other emergencies also impact on mental health and psychosocial wellbeing (Tol et al., 2013; International Committee

of the Red Cross, 2021), with an estimated 1 in 5 persons in conflict-affected communities living with a mental health condition, ranging from mild depression to more intense symptoms such as post-traumatic stress and post-traumatic stress disorder (International Committee of the Red Cross, 2021).

When the National Health Service (NHS) was first established in the United Kingdom (UK) in 1948 it focused, similar to other global healthcare systems at the time, on treating single conditions or illnesses (Foucault, 1973). This approach inadequately reflects the multi-dimensional nature of mental health and the complex interplay of psychosocial, environmental, biological, and genetic factors across the life course as they impact the experiences of the people affected (Thornton, 2019).

In recent decades. health and care needs have become increasingly more complex with people living longer and requiring protracted support from many different services and professionals (King's Fund, 2022). The public health white paper, *Healthy Lives, Healthy People* (Department of Health and Social Care, 2010), was one of the first public health strategies to give equal weight to both mental and physical health. In addition, the cross-government mental health outcomes strategy on *No Health without Mental Health*, *NHS Five Year Forward View, Long Term Plan*, and *Mental Health Implementation Plan* (Department of Health and Social Care, 2011; NHS, 2014, 2019a, 2019b) outlined mental health as a priority and vowed to work towards a future that removes the divide between physical and mental health. From a global perspective, the example of mental health and substance use as targets within the health sustainable development goals (United Nations, 2015), as well as a global shortage of mental health practitioners (International Council of Nurses, 2022), reflect a transformative vision to reframe the worldwide mental health agenda.

Despite these important milestones, access to timely, integrated, and appropriate mental health care remain a work-in-progress with people too often receiving fragmented care from services that are not effectively supported or co-ordinated around an individual's needs (Royal College of Psychiatrists, 2019; King's Fund, 2022). The title of this pillar – no health without mental health – is underpinned by a commitment to mental health as a fundamental human right, crucial to personal, community and socioeconomic development. To further exemplify this point, in the next section, readers are introduced to an anonymised scenario based on Matthew's experiences of mental and physical health difficulties. The discussion which follows demonstrates the relevance, benefit, importance, and necessity of a holistic approach.

Application of No Health without Mental Health Pillar to Scenario

The purpose of the following is to highlight how mental health intersects with other needs, demonstrating the importance to reflect on these links to ensure holistic care. Williamson et al. (2019) identified that musculoskeletal injury is the most common cause of medical discharge from the army. The impact of the shoulder injury is significant not only due to the ongoing physical challenges, including long term pain and impact on sleep, but also the psychological and social toll on Matthew's life.

Early discharge from the military, while learning to navigate the transition and attempting to cope with the physical and/or mental strain (resulting in medical discharge) can be a challenging time for veterans (Holliday and Pedersen, 2017). A medical and unplanned discharge from the military, is associated with hardships, including financial stress, as well as the potential for experiencing loneliness and challenges adjusting to a new routine (Burdett et al., 2019; Guthrie-Gower and Wilson-Menzfeld, 2022; Armed Forces Covenant Fund Trust, 2022). Furthermore, research suggests this type of injury, and the level of pain experienced, are strong risk factors for mental health difficulties (Sareen et al., 2013).

The research cited above resonates with Matthew's experiences. Matthew was proud of his army career, and valued his time in the armed forces as it gave him structure, friendships, an active lifestyle as well as meaning and dignity to his life. Since losing his military career, Matthew no longer engages in activities that bring him joy. He has seen his marriage break down resulting in little access to his children, has struggled to maintain a job and is living an increasingly isolated lifestyle. Losing elements of an individual's identity can profoundly impact on mental health. According to Charmaz (1983), the loss of self is a form of suffering, resulting in a psychological distress, increasing an isolated life and feelings of grief, alongside seeing oneself as an inconvenience to others, and uncertainty about what the future holds (Boss, 1999). Losing a sense of self affects many areas of meaningful living, represented by Matthew questioning 'what is left for him in life', as well as the disruption to his sleep caused by pain, which he attempts to mitigate through alcohol use.

Matthew presents with further factors that shape, compound and exacerbate his current health status. For example, Matthew is a cisgender male in his early forties, a father and an army veteran who is experiencing chronic pain – all factors identified as a correlative risk for experiences of mental ill health (Burdett et al., 2019; Samaritans, 2017; Mind, 2020; Stiawa et al., 2020; Office for Health Improvements and Disparities, 2021a). It is widely recognised that the notion that 'being male' can be associated with individual's reluctance to seek support for their mental health, often intersected with the perception of stigma around discussing mental health difficulties (Sharp et al., 2022). Nevertheless, the prevalence of male mental distress, involving feeling worried or low in mood has doubled to the rate of women over the last decade (Mind, 2020).

Amid the adjustment to a new way of life involving social isolation and impaired sleep, Matthew is also experiencing chronic pain. Pain is described as an unpleasant sensory and emotional experience associated with actual or potential tissue damage (Treede, 2018). As pain becomes chronic, there is functional reorganisation and changes in neural connectivity, where processing of all pain shifts to the limbic system of the brain, involved in behavioural and emotional responses (Apkarian et al., 2011; Baliki et al., 2012). Across diverse aetiologies, the brain of the person with chronic pain shows consistent functional, structural, and molecular changes, as well as an impact on mood and deficits in attention, memory, learning, decision making and impulsivity (Khera and Rangasamy, 2021). While reversible with treatment, the pain Matthew is experiencing is not being managed, bringing about ongoing mental distress and mobility difficulties. This is exemplified through Matthew's current use of alcohol to manage the pain and aid sleep, both of which are a physical and mental health concern. In the short-term alcohol may help falling asleep, as well as reduce inhibitions, and tensions about self-consciousness. However long-term physical effects of alcohol have a detrimental impact on an individual's quality of life. This includes the risk of increased blood pressure, gastric ulcers, acid reflux and impairing circadian rhythms (natural changes regulating the sleep–wake cycle approximately every 24 hours) (Colrain, Nicholas, and Baker, 2014; Scott, Aboud and Smith, 2022; Scott et al., 2021; Office for Health Improvements and Disparities, 2021b).

While the link between alcohol and diabetes is still under study, alcohol is high in calories increasing hunger and satiation, escalating calorie consumption, and weight gain (Kim and Kim, 2012). Alcohol intake also potentially increases weight, with weight gain being a significant risk factor with developing type 2 diabetes (Wilding, 2014). Matthew's impaired sleep may also affect his weight, compounding his low mood perhaps around body image, and increasing hunger (for energy to remain awake) leading to further calorie consumption (Papatriantafyllou et al., 2022). Alcohol also affects mental health, such as increasing the risk of self-harm and suicide as well as experiencing depression and anxiety, alongside social difficulties, among which involve arguments whether with family, friends and/or work colleagues (Sullivan, Fiellin, and O'Connor, 2005; McIntosh and Ritson, 2001). Therefore, healthcare professionals should be aware of the pertinent losses to Matthew's identity, and factors such as financial issues owing to unemployment, social isolation, alcohol use and history (notably ACES), as accumulatively, these increase the likelihood of mental ill health and experiencing suicidal ideation (Oexle et al., 2018; Fryers and Brugha, 2013).

Although physical injuries and chronic health conditions can, and should, be treated, it is important to remember that these conditions are part of a wider 'self'. Treatment and care should always be given with a comprehensive view of the potential impact these health issues can have on an individual. Professionals need to broaden their horizon around the potential for these to cause or exacerbate difficulties associated with health.

Dualism, Holism, and Stress Vulnerability

The above scenario and research highlights that treating physical ill health solely is no longer in line with the evidence base, and this evidence does not support adopting a singular model of disease. Therefore, it is necessary to consider a wider and holistic picture when working with patients in the provision of optimum nursing care.

Smuts (1926), who coined the term 'holism', argues that the term encapsulates and addresses how individuals intersect with aspects of the self and their environment, further developed by Engel (1977) with the biopsychosocial model, explored in the recovery section below. Its philosophical underpinnings, however, appear to stem from ancient Indian Vedic culture (*c.*1500–500 BC), with the 'sarvah' vernacular, denoting a person within the universe (Erickson, 2007). While such philosophical reflection might seem immaterial, the universe in the scenario, include factors that constitutes Matthew's life, such as mental, physical, and psychological health needs. Moreover, recovery, as will be further outlined, aims to enrich meaningfulness to life with needs also situated culturally, socially, and historically, such as spiritual requisites and what Matthew believes historically led to his current difficulties, including what the scenario refers to as a 'difficult upbringing' (Chidarikire, 2012).

Reductionism, which contributes to diminishing whole persons to specific biological parts, needs to be challenged and is not in keeping with the 'no health without mental health' principle which values holism. This is impacted by dualism – a view that the mind and body are separate entities. The philosopher René Descartes (2003 [1641]) argued that the body and mind function independently, in that unlike the mind, the body cannot think, and thinking is of a higher value in terms of ourselves, represented by the principle of 'I think therefore I am'. As much research attests, it is not merely that one difficulty occurs in isolation from others and should be considered as part of a wider 'self', wider systems, and cultures. Further challenges might involve challenging a biomedical focus, where care is reactive rather than preventative and directed towards recovery. Meeting the complex needs associated with holism requires engagement with wider social factors such as social inequalities which impact health and wellbeing (Foucault, 1973). Such factors impact Matthew's scenario and, perhaps, the significance of veteran versus civilian identities in relation to the experience of mental distress.

With the stress vulnerability model, stressful life events increase the likelihood of illness (Zubin and Spring, 1977). This can establish wide ranging holistic factors around illnesses generally, but not at the exclusion of mental health needs. We see recovery integral to holism, whereby difficulties such as loss of identities, feeling hopeless and worthless, are not only factors increasing alcohol consumption and risk of type 2 diabetes. Equally important are the stress factors resulting in hopelessness, without which, Matthew might not be drinking so heavily. The stress vulnerability model purports that while genetics increase vulnerability, it is the life stressors – such as the breakdown of Matthew's marriage and disconnection from his children – which increase the likelihood of ill-health (Anderson, Ramo, and Brown, 2006). These factors are intrinsically related to mental health, for example, thwarted belongingness contributes to mental distress, while absence of meaningful support increases stress vulnerability, markedly with Matthew appearing to use alcohol to mitigate troubling feelings (Scott, Aboud, and Smith, 2022).

Questions might arise why people make 'choices', which from an observer perspective, appear to obviously impact negatively on their lives. In terms of holism, it is important to recognise that when experiencing mental distress, choices are not so obvious, with one reason being by how the body reacts to mental and psychological stress, termed fight, flight, or freeze (Llera, Newman, and Michelle, 2020). Essentially the nervous system is in 'survival mode' to cope resulting in tunnel vision, limiting abilities to see how problems could be resolved, and even why these problems exist. Care options in such situations can include exploring motivation for change, that is, what might lessen drinking for example (Latchford and Duff, 2010). Reasons to change are not dictated by the nurse, for like most people, being told what to do can be the antithesis for change, requiring a collaborative approach to what change will add to Matthew's life. Matthew might point out that alcohol use results in having hangovers impeding abilities to do things he feels are important, and for a fuller account in how motivational approaches might assist, a link is available with the above citation in the reference list, about what such a motivational approach might entail.

In terms of the stress vulnerability model, Matthew might not yet realise why life is difficult. Hence, a starting point is to explore stress factors making life difficult and the reasons why, to inform holistic care interventions. While standardised assessments are commonplace to gather such information, as discussed in the patient involvement chapter, the use of art-based interventions have merit, and we recommend the stress beaker, in recognition that the kinaesthetic-tactile qualities of 'doing', may ground a person, and transverse some tunnel vision owing to distress (Neha and Tamplin, 2022). By Matthew and the nurse filling in a beaker literally drawn on paper, the beaker becomes a metaphor, and water drops falling into the beaker represent life stressors (Brabban and Turkington, 2002).

Through water levels rising with each stressful event, Matthew may see that when the water overfills, symbolises a tipping point to perhaps where Matthew is now. Moreover, a tap can be figuratively attached to the beaker, exploring what might lessen the water level. Whereas such approaches are the tip of the iceberg in what holism may provide, it may begin to sketch a recovery pathway, one which Matthew finds personally meaningful, and perhaps more likely to succeed, given Matthew is seen as a whole person rather than just one or two conditions. The points raised show mental health care is an area of overall health, rather than sitting outside of it, which continues to develop, grow, and challenge researchers to this day.

Holism, Coordination, and Recovery-Focused Care

As highlighted, nursing care aims to be holistic, enriching personal agency to have a fulfilling life and focussing on all care needs, as discussed in Fundamentals of Care chapter. In terms of Matthew, an integrated approach is required that encapsulates his care with equity, exemplified by incorporating Matthew's voice with making choices about his treatment, and addressing Matthew as a whole person, not separated into components (Castillo et al., 2019). Healthcare services can be split by the nature of provision, thus creating a dualism or divide between physical health and mental health services, as well as the divide between health and social care (Naylor et al., 2016). While fully integrated care systems (unifying different health and social care services together) may not entirely resolve the provision of care due to the nuances of individual healthcare needs; a more collaborative approach may seek to reduce the disruption faced by individuals in accessing care.

The NHS *Five Year Forward View for Mental Health* (NHS, 2014) anticipated a trajectory to increase the community mental health care provision as a recovery-focussed alternative to inpatient mental health care. Recovery focussed care is whereby a person is supported to have a meaningful life despite experiencing mental health difficulties (Anthony, 1993). Moreover, it aims to focus on empowering individuals regarding their specific aspirations and goals rather than only focusing the goals of clinicians that tend to involve the mitigation of illness (Simpson et al., 2016). Hence rather than a combatant distinction, sometimes referred to the personal recovery versus clinical recovery, care aims to involve collaboration in which the expertise of the patient and their significant others work alongside the expertise of clinicians (Macpherson et al., 2016). In this context, Matthew's care is likely coordinated by one named professional within a mental health team as seen in Europe and Oceania (Banfield et al., 2012). A care coordinator's role is to liaise with other teams or multi-professional members to ensure collaborative and holistic working alongside the individual, as well as a central point of contact for the individual, their significant others and service providers (National Institute for Health and Care Excellence, 2018, 2019). Similarly, to other international services, such coordination stems from a Community Mental Health Team within the UK, given their vantage point of Matthew's care and consistency of involvement (Simpson et al., 2016).

The role of a Community Mental Health Team particular in western countries, is to provide ongoing assessment, review, and support of individual's health care needs, predominantly focussing on recovery focussed care planning, risk assessment involving but not limited to risks such as suicide and management within the community setting. This may also result in input from other professionals, dependent on needs. For example, in Matthew's case, a substance misuse services may be included (for his alcohol consumption and associated feelings around his use), as well as veteran mental health services, local doctor, chronic pain teams, charity organisations to name a few. Matthew's care coordinator can also support Matthew in ensuring his accommodation is secure, aid with seeking employment, alongside access to financial support organisations and any other social care assistance needed. By collaboratively working to support individuals from different specialist areas, it can help to ensure that Matthew's physical and mental health is reviewed and assessed holistically, and that he feels wholly supported. Hence it benefits that coordinators have in-depth knowledge of the locality that they serve so it can be adopted as a resource to improve Matthew's mental health (NHS England and NHS Improvement and the National Collaborating Central for Mental Health, 2019).

Included as a community resource are charities (or third sector organisations), which can also help to provide support with social/lifestyle aspects that may benefit Matthew in finding new friendships, activities, peer support (support from a person with shared experiences) and purpose. Another important consideration is Matthew's military experiences and significance with his current mental health experiences. Sharing time and narratives with groups of people who are also veterans, and experienced medical discharge, can be helpful in Matthew gaining a sense of being seen, heard, and understood, and likely to enrich more meaningful support and a sense of healing (Meyerson et al., 2022; Regel and Joseph, 2017; Boss, 1999). Offers of linking Matthew with such services should be conducted with transparency, and in collaboration to ensure, as recovery focused practices attest, that the support provided focuses on the areas Matthew would like to address and the approach is meaningful to Matthew's life (Kelly et al., 2019).

The biopsychosocial approach as first illustrated above was developed by Dr George Engel in 1977 – it is a seminal model that explores the biological, psychological, and social aspects of individuals' health (Engel, 1977) and can be utilised as part of recovery to assess and plan care focussed around external and internal processes of a person (McKay et al., 2012). The model integrates the consideration of genetics, socioeconomic status, psychological coping mechanisms among other factors, to help individuals and healthcare professionals to cultivate meanings with patients around personal experiences and collaboratively pinpoint areas of focus (McKay et al., 2012). With Matthew, we would see emerging factors in each biopsychosocial area of the model whereby care could be identified and coordinated according to his experience of chronic pain, psychological trauma in the military and relationship difficulties. The combination of considering these factors, while identifying Matthew's personal goals, will frame plans around his recovery journey in which understanding about attaining personal needs may grow overtime (Griffiths and Ryan, 2008).

The recovery approach is individual to each person and considers their goals, expectations and wishes for their future. This is guided, assessed, and supported by healthcare professionals to achieve their potential, while acknowledging that 'cure' does not have to be present for individuals to experience fulfilment (Coffey et al., 2019). It is a framework that encapsulates all factors identified in the biopsychosocial model (Engel, 1977), and encourages empowerment and self-advocacy by allowing full engagement and collaboration between mental health services and individuals. Matthew's goals may range from receiving further treatment for his shoulder injury, effective pain management and getting back to a fitness to play rugby as he previously enjoyed, to reducing his alcohol intake with support and/or to be able to reconnect with his children and improve his daily mood/mental state. Healthcare professionals can consider the interplaying of biopsychosocial factors to develop a recovery focussed care plan for Matthew that equally considers his physical and mental health recovery, all of which are interdependent to some extent.

Similarly, to the above, particularly in terms of fractured service provision, is the frustration associated with a lack of integrated electronic patient record systems, cited as a significant contributing factor to delaying care for individuals (Ser, Robertson, and Sheikh, 2014). While it may be argued that such split in service provision exists to champion clinical specialities and empower health and social care professionals to thrive within their scope of practice, the negative impact on the coherent provision of holistic care is undeniable. As discussed with 'siloing' above regarding holism and rendering individuals to mere physical or mental health symptoms, it undermines the multifaceted nature of humanity and downplays how the physiological, psychological, and social needs, to name a few, intersect as well as obscuring abilities to understand the entire needs of a person. Also worth noting is that human interaction has the potential to be an intervention, and can afford safety, enhance stability, and promote recovery. Herman (1992) speaks to the importance of relationships when discussing recovery, emphasising recovery can only take place in the context of thoughtful interactions and therapeutic relationships. A care coordinator can work to create culture that promotes safety (including physical, relational, moral, and emotional). This is while recognise asymmetrical power and give patients a robust voice with decision-making, to ensure, when possible, that the care provided resonates with the holistic needs of the person.

Conclusion

Throughout history understanding mental health difficulties. as experienced by Mathew in the scenario, can be linked with degrees of misunderstanding. Yet, progress does exist, illustrated by holism, recovery, and person centeredness in the chapter. Researching the origins and manifestation of mental distress is ongoing, gaining understanding from the intimate, connections between the mind and body, while individuals living with mental ill health learn to cultivate ways, ideally with the support from others, to live fulfilling lives despite experiencing difficulties. Nevertheless, ethical, and philosophical challenges somewhat continue around integrating multifaceted concepts, notably bringing together biological and psychosocial factors into patient care. This is without losing sight that such care requires to be meaningful and attuned to the sensitivities of the human condition.

Takeaways for Student Nurses

- Mental health is an intrinsic part of our individual and collective health and well-being (World Health Organization, 2022).
- It is important to recognise that there is value in checking the physical health status of a patient, as well as their mental health. Social factors also play a major role in determining the mental health status of individuals, interacting with more proximal genetic factors and individual experiences across the life course (Connell, O'Cathain, and Brazier, 2014).
- There is a need to expand our understanding of mental health from the existing focus on clinically defined mental disorders to a broader dimensional approach to mental health (Alegría et al., 2018).
- Tackling social determinants of mental health is likely to require the coordination of a range of social, health, education, and the justice sector (Alegría et al., 2018).
- Mental health is a universal and basic human right. From a social justice perspective, this emphasises the rights of populations (such as those fleeing conflict),

who are at increased risk of developing mental distress, as well as the rights of people already living with mental health difficulties (Mann, Bradley, and Sahakian, 2016).

Takeaways for Educators/Practitioners

- The professional, institutional, and cultural separation of mental and physical health creates substantial costs for both patients and the health system. Through an integrated response to the multiple needs of patients, there is scope to reduce these costs while improving quality of care (Naylor et al., 2016).
- As policymakers and professionals increasingly focus on how integrated care can become a reality, integration of mental and physical health care must become a key part of the debate (Naylor et al., 2016).
- There is a need for alignment of evidence from diverse fields, including the genetic, developmental, social, and biological determinants of mental health (Naylor et al., 2016).
- With a better understanding of social determinants, population-level interventions that target these determinants can be planned more effectively and efficiently, helping to address health inequalities (Alegría et al., 2018).
- With the large body of international research and policy regarding the UN Millennium Development Goals, and recently, sustainable development goals, it is essential to link mental health with international development targets (Tol et al., 2013).

References

Alegría, M., NeMoyer, A., Falgàs Bagué, I., Wang, Y. and Alvarez, K. (2018) 'Social determinants of mental health: where we are and where we need to go', *Current Psychiatry Reports*, 20, pp. 1–13.

Alloh, F.T., Regmi, P., Onche, I., van Teijlingen, E. and Trenoweth, S., 2018. 'Mental Health in low-and middle income countries (LMICs): Going beyond the need for funding', *Health Prospect: Journal of Public Health*, 17(1), pp. 12–17.

Anderson, K.G., Ramo, D.E. and Brown, S.A. (2006) 'Life stress, coping and comorbid youth: An examination of the stress-vulnerability model for substance relapse', *Journal of Psychoactive Drugs*, 38(3), pp. 255–262.

Anthony, W.A. (1993) 'Recovery from mental illness: The guiding vision of the mental health service system in the 1990s', *Psychosocial Rehabilitation Journal*, 16(4), pp. 11–23.

Apkarian V. A., Hashmi, J. A. and Baliki, M. N. (2011) 'Pain and the brain: specificity and plasticity of the brain in clinical chronic pain', *Pain*, 152(3 Suppl), pp. 1–35.

Armed Forces Covenant Fund Trust. (2022) 'Evaluation report for tackling loneliness'. Available at: https://covenantfund.org.uk/resources/e valuation-report-for-tackling-loneliness/ (Accessed: 12 April 2023).

Ashton, K., Bellis, M. and Hughes, K. (2016a) 'Adverse childhood experiences and their association with health-harming behaviours and mental wellbeing in the Welsh adult population: a national cross-sectional survey', *The Lancet*, 388, p. S21.

Ashton, K., Bellis, M. A., Davis, A.R., Hardcastle, K., and Hughes, K. (2016b) 'Adverse childhood experiences and their association with chronic disease and health service use in the Welsh adult population'. Available at: www.basw.co.uk/resources/adverse-childhood-experiences-and-their-association-chronic-disease-and-health-service-use (Accessed: 11 April 2023).

Baliki, M.N., Petre, B., Torbey, S., Herrmann, K.M., Huang, L., Schnitzer, T.J., Fields, H.L., and Apkarian, A.V. (2012) 'Corticostriatal functional connectivity predicts transition to chronic back pain', *Nature Neuroscience*, 15(8), pp. 1117–1119.

Banfield, M. A., Gardner, K.L., Yen, L.E., McRae, I.S., Gillespie, J.A. and Wells, R.W. (2012) 'Coordination of care in Australian mental health policy', *Australian Health Review*, 36(2), pp. 153–157.

Barnett, K., Mercer, S.W., Norbury, M., Watt, G., Wyke, S. and Guthrie, B. (2012) 'Epidemiology of multimorbidity and implications for health care, research, and medical education: a cross-sectional study', *The Lancet*, 380(9836), pp. 37–43.

Bellis, M., Hughes, K., Ford, K., Rodriguez, G. R., Sethi, D. and Passmore, J. (2019) 'Life course health consequences and associated annual costs of adverse childhood experiences across Europe and North America: a systematic review and meta-analysis', *The Lancet Public Health*, 4(10), pp. 1–12.

Boss, P. (1999) *Ambiguous Loss. Learning to Live with Unresolved Grief.* Cambridge, MA: Harvard University Press.

Brabban, A. and Turkington, D. (2002) 'The Search for Meaning: detecting congruence between life events, underlying schema and psychotic symptoms', in A.P. Morrison (ed.), A *Casebook of Cognitive Therapy for Psychosis*. New York: Brunner-Routledge, pp. 59–75.

Brown, D.W., Anda, R.F., Tiemeier, H., Felitti, V.J., Edwards, V.J., Croft, J.B. and Giles, W.H. (2009) 'Adverse childhood experiences and the risk of premature mortality', *American Journal of Preventive Medicine*, 37(5), pp. 389–396.

Burdett, H., Fear, N.T., MacManus, D., Wessely, S., Rona, R.J. and Greenberg, N. (2019) 'Unemployment and benefit claims by UK veterans in the new millennium: results from a record linkage study', *Occupational and Environmental Medicine*, 76(10), pp. 726–732.

Castillo, E.G., Ijadi-Maghsoodi, R., Shadravan, S., Moore, E., Mensah, M.O., Docherty, M., Aguilera Nunez, M.G., Barcelo, N., Goodsmith, N., Halpin, L.E. and Morton, I. (2019) 'Community interventions to promote mental health and social equity', *Current Psychiatry Reports*, 21, pp. 1–14.

Charmaz, K. (1983) 'Loss of self: a fundamental form of suffering in the chronically ill', *Sociology of Health and Illness*, 5(2), pp. 168–195.

Chidarikire. S (2012) 'Spirituality: The neglected dimension of holistic mental health care', *Advances in Mental Health,* 10(3), pp. 298–302.

Coffey, M., Hannigan, B., Barlow, S., Cartwright, M., Cohen, R., Faulkner, A., Jones, A. and Simpson, A. (2019) 'Recovery-focused mental health care planning and co-ordination in acute inpatient mental health settings: a cross national comparative mixed methods study', *BMC Psychiatry*, 19(1), pp. 1–18.

Colrain, I.M., Nicholas, C.L. and Baker, F.C. (2014) 'Alcohol and the sleeping brain', *Handbook of Clinical Neurology*, 125, pp. 415–431.

Connell, J., O'Cathain, A. and Brazier, J. (2014) 'Measuring quality of life in mental health: are we asking the right questions?' *Social Science and Medicine*, 120, pp. 12–20.

Department of Health and Social Care (2010) 'Healthy lives, healthy people: Our strategy for public department of health in England'. Available at: https://webarchive.nationalarchives.gov.uk/ukgwa/20130107105354/www.dh.gov.uk/prod_consum_dh/groups/dh_digitalassets/@dh/@en/@ps/documents/digitalasset/dh_122347.pdf (Accessed: 12 April 2023).

Department of Health and Social Care (2011) 'No health without mental health: A cross-government outcomes strategy'. Available at: www.gov.uk/government/publications/no-health-without-mental-health-a-cross-government-outcomes-strategy (Accessed: 12 April 2023).

Descartes, R. (2003 [1641]) *Meditations and Other Metaphysical Writings*. London: Penguin Publishing.

Engel, G. L. (1977) 'The need for a new medical model: a challenge for biomedicine', *Science,* 196(4286), pp. 129–136.

Erickson. H. L (2007) 'Philosophy and Theory of Holism', *The Nursing Clinics of North America,* 42(2), pp. 139–163.

Foucault, M. (1973) *The Birth of the Clinic: An Archaeology of Medical Perception.* London: Tavistock Publications Limited.

Fryers, T. and Brugha, T. (2013) 'Childhood determinants of adult psychiatric disorder. Clinical practice and epidemiology in mental health', *Clinical Practice and Epidemiology in Mental Health,* 9, pp. 1–50.

Griffiths, C.A. and Ryan, P. (2008) 'Recovery and Lifelong Learning: Interrelated Processes', *International Journal of Psychosocial Rehabilitation,* 13(1), pp. 51–56.

Guthrie-Gower, S. and Wilson-Menzfeld, G. (2022) 'Ex-military personnel's experiences of loneliness and social isolation from discharge, through transition, to the present day', *PloS one,* 17(6), pp. 1–17.

Herman, J. (1992) *Trauma and Recovery: The Aftermath of Violence – From Domestic Abuse to Political Terror.* New York: Basic Books.

Holliday, S.B. and Pedersen, E.R. (2017) 'The association between discharge status, mental health, and substance misuse among young adult veterans', *Psychiatry Research,* 256, pp. 428–434.

Hughes, K., Bellis, M.A., Hardcastle, K.A., Sethi, D., Butchart, A., Mikton, C., Jones, L. and Dunne, M.P. (2017) 'The effect of multiple adverse childhood experiences on health: a systematic review and meta-analysis', *Lancet Public Health,* 2(8) pp. 356–366.

International Committee of the Red Cross. (2021) 'Mental health and psychosocial support'. Available at: www.icrc.org/en/what-we-do/health/mental-health (Accessed: 12 April 2023).

International Council of Nurses. (2022) 'The global mental health nursing workforce: Time to prioritize and invest in mental health and wellbeing'. Available at: www.icn.ch/sites/default/files/inline-files/ICN_Mental_Health_Workforce_ report_EN_web.pdf (Accessed: 13 April 2023).

Kelly, D., Steiner, A., Mason, H. and Teasdale, S. (2019) 'Men's Sheds: A conceptual exploration of the causal pathways for health and well-being', *Health and Social Care in the Community,* 27(5), pp. 1147–1157.

Khera, T. and Rangasamy, V. (2021) 'Cognition and pain: a review', *Frontiers in Psychology,* 12, pp. 1–11.

Kim, S. J. and Kim, D. J. (2012) 'Alcoholism and diabetes mellitus', *Diabetes and Metabolism Journal,* 36(2), pp. 108–115.

King's Fund. (2012) 'Long term conditions and mental health: The cost of comorbidities'. Available at: www.kingsfund.org.uk/sites/default/files/field/field_publication_file/long-term-conditions-mental-health-cost-comorbidities-naylor-feb12.pdf (Accessed: 12 April 2023).

King's Fund. (2022) 'Integrated care systems explained'. Available at: www.kingsfund.org.uk/publications/integrated-care-systems-explained#:~:text=As%20a%20consequence%2C%20people%20too,and%20create%20duplication%20and%20inefficiency (Accessed: 12 April 2023).

Lancet Global Health. (2020) 'Editorial: Mental health matters'. Available at: www.thelancet.com/action/showPdf?pii=S2214-109X%2820%2930432-0 (Accessed 11 April 2023).

Latchford, G. and Duff, A. (2010) Motivational interviewing: A brief guide. Available at: CF MI guide 2010.pdf (swswchd.co.uk) (Accessed: 12 February 2023).

Liu, N.H., Daumit, G.L., Dua, T., Aquila, R., Charlson, F., Cuijpers, P., Druss, B., Dudek, K., Freeman, M., Fujii, C. and Gaebel, W., 2017. Excess mortality in persons with severe mental disorders: a multilevel intervention framework and priorities for clinical practice, policy and research agendas. *World Psychiatry,* 16(1), pp. 30–40.

Llera, S. J. and Newman. M. G. (2020) 'Worry impairs the problem-solving process: Results from an experimental study', *Behaviour Research and Therapy,* 135, pp. 103759–103759.

Macpherson, R., Pesola, F., Leamy, M., Bird, V., Le Boutillier, C., Williams, J. and Slade, M. (2016) 'The relationship between clinical and recovery dimensions of outcome in mental health', *Schizophrenia Research,* 175(1–3), pp. 142–147.

Mahomed, F. (2020) Addressing the problem of severe underinvestment in mental health and well-being from a human rights perspective. Health and human rights, 22(1), pp. 35–49.

Mann, S.P., Bradley, V.J. and Sahakian, B.J. (2016) 'Human rights-based approaches to mental health: a review of programs', *Health and Human Rights*, 18(1), pp. 263–275.

Maté, G. and Maté, D. (2022) *The Myth of Normal: Trauma, Illness and Healing in a Toxic Culture*. New York: Random House.

McIntosh, C. and Ritson, B. (2001) 'Treating depression complicated by substance misuse', *Advances in Psychiatric Treatment*, 7(5), pp. 357–364.

McKay, R., McDonald, R., Lie, D. and McGowan, H. (2012) 'Reclaiming the best of the biopsychosocial model of mental health care and 'recovery' for older people through a 'person-centred' approach', *Australasian Psychiatry*, 20(6), pp. 492–495.

Meyerson, J.L., O'Malley, K.A., Obas, C.E. and Hinrichs, K.L. (2022) 'Lived Experience: A Case-Based Review of Trauma-Informed Hospice and Palliative Care at a Veterans Affairs Medical Center', *American Journal of Hospice and Palliative Medicine*, 40(3), pp. 329–336.

Mind. (2020) 'Get it off your chest: Men's mental health 10 years on'. Available at: www.mind.org.uk/media/6771/get-it-off-your-chest_a4_final.pdf (Accessed: 24 January 2023).

Naito, R., Leong, D.P., Bangdiwala, S.I., McKee, M., Subramanian, S.V., Rangarajan, S., Islam, S., Avezum, A., Yeates, K.E., Lear, S.A. and Gupta, R. (2021) 'Impact of social isolation on mortality and morbidity in 20 high-income, middle-income and low-income countries in five continents', *BMJ Global Health*, 6(3), pp. 1–11.

National Institute of Mental Health (2021) 'Chronic illness and mental health: Recognising and treating depression'. Available at: www.nimh.nih.gov/health/publications/chronic-illness-mental-health (Accessed: 12 April 2023).

NHS. (2014) 'Five year forward view'. Available at: www.england.nhs.uk/wp-content/uploads/2014/10/5yfv-web.pdf (Accessed: 12 April 2023).

NHS. (2019a) 'Long term plan'. Available at: www.longtermplan.nhs.uk/ (Accessed: 12 April 2023).

NHS. (2019b) 'Mental health implementation plan 2019/20–2023/24'. Available at: www.longtermplan.nhs.uk/publication/nhs-mental-health-implementation-plan-2019-20-2023-24/ (Accessed: 12 April 2023).

NHS England and NHS Improvement and the National Collaborating Central for Mental Health. (2019) 'The community mental health framework for adults and older adults'. Available at: www.england.nhs.uk/wp-content/uploads/2019/09/community-mental-health-framework-for-adults-and-older-adults.pdf (Accessed: 11 April 2023).

National Institute for Health and Care Excellence. (2018) 'Mental health and the national health service: what's changed and what's to come?' Available at: https://indepth.nice.org.uk/mental-health-and-the-nhs/index.html (Accessed: 12 April 2023).

National Institute for Health and Care Excellence. (2019) 'Coexisting severe mental illness and substance misuse: Quality standard [QS188]'. Available at: www.nice.org.uk/guidance/qs188/chapter/quality-statement-3-care-coordinators (Accessed: 31 January 2023).

Naylor, C., Parsonage, M., McDaid, D., Knapp, M., Fossey, M. Galea, A. (2012) 'Long-term conditions and mental health: The cost of co-morbidities'. Available at: www.kingsfund.org.uk/sites/default/files/field/field_publication_file/long-term-conditions-mental-health-cost-comorbidities-naylor-feb12.pdf (Accessed: 31 January 2023).

Naylor, C., Das, P., Ross, S., Honeyman, M., Thompson, J. and Gilburt, H. (2016) 'Bringing together physical and mental health: A new frontier for integrated care'. Available at: www.basw.co.uk/system/files/resources/basw_101420-2_0.pdf (Accessed: 9 March 2023)

Neha, C. and Tamplin, J. (2022) 'The Use of Kinesthetic Empathy with Adults Living with Treatment Resistant Depression: A Survey Study', *American Journal of Dance Therapy*, 44(2), pp. 115–142.

Oexle, N., Waldmann, T., Staiger, T., Xu, Z. and Rüsch, N. (2018) 'Mental illness stigma and suicidality: the role of public and individual stigma', *Epidemiology and Psychiatric Sciences*, 27(2), pp. 169–175.

Office for Health Improvements and Disparities. (2021a) 'COVID-19 mental health and wellbeing surveillance: Spotlights'. Available at: www.gov.uk/government/publications/covid-19-mental-health-and-wellbeing-surveillance-spotlights (Accessed: 9 March 2023).

Office for Health Improvements and Disparities. (2021b) 'Chapter 12: Alcohol'. Available at: www.gov.uk/government/publications/delivering-better-oral-health-an-evidence-based-toolkit-for-prevention/chapter-12-alcohol#fn:7 (Accessed: 9 March 2023).

Office for Health Improvements and Disparities. (2023) 'Premature mortality in adults with severe mental illness'. Available at: www.gov.uk/government/publications/premature-mortality-in-adults-with-severe-mental-illness/premature-mortality-in-adults-with-severe-mental-illness-smi#main-findings (Accessed: 9 March 2023).

Organisation for Economic Co-operation and Development Stat. (2021) Health expenditure and financing. Available at: https://stats.oecd.org/Index.aspx?DataSetCode=SHA (Accessed: 13 April 2023)

Papatriantafyllou, E., Efthymiou, D., Zoumbaneas, E., Popescu, C.A. and Vassilopoulou, E. (2022) 'Sleep Deprivation: Effects on Weight Loss and Weight Loss Maintenance', *Nutrients*, 14(8), pp. 1549–1562.

Patel, V., Saxena, S., Lund, C., Thornicroft, G., Baingana, F., Bolton, P., Chisholm, D., Collins, P.Y., Cooper, J.L., Eaton, J. and Herrman, H. (2018) 'The Lancet Commission on global mental health and sustainable development', *The Lancet*, 392(10157), pp. 1553–1598.

Pedersen, K. M. (2019) 'The Nordic health care systems: Most similar comparative research?' *Nordic Journal of Health Economics*, 6(2), pp. 99–107.

Public Health England. (2018) 'Severe mental illness and physical health inequalities: briefing'. Available at: www.gov.uk/government/publications/severe-mental-illness-smi-physical-health-inequalities/severe-mental-illness-and-physical-health-inequalities-briefing (Accessed: 9 March 2023).

Rajkumar, R. P. (2022) 'The Correlates of Government Expenditure on Mental Health Services: An Analysis of Data From 78 Countries and Regions; *Cureus*, 14(8). pp. 1–11.

Rathod, S., Pinninti, N., Irfan, M., Gorczynski, P., Rathod, P., Gega, L. and Naeem, F. (2017) 'Mental health service provision in low-and middle-income countries' *Health Services Insights*, 10, pp. 1–7.

Regel, S. and Joseph, S. (2017) *Post-Traumatic Stress: The Facts*. Oxford: Oxford University Press.

Rennick-Egglestone, S., Ramsay, A., McGranahan, R., Llewellyn-Beardsley, J., Hui, A., Pollock, K., Repper, J., Yeo, C., Ng, F., Roe, J., Gillard, S., Thornicroft, G., Booth, S. and Slade, M. (2019) 'The impact of mental health recovery narratives on recipients experiencing mental health problems: Qualitative analysis and change model', *PLoS One*, 14(12), pp. 1–23.

Ronaldson, A., de la Torre, J.A., Prina, M., Armstrong, D., Das-Munshi, J., Hatch, S., Stewart, R., Hotopf, M. and Dregan, A. (2021) 'Associations between physical multimorbidity patterns and common mental health disorders in middle-aged adults: A prospective analysis using data from the UK Biobank', *The Lancet Regional Health-Europe*, 8, pp. 1–12.

Royal College of Psychiatrists. (2019) 'Improving mental health services in systems of integrated and accountable care: emerging lessons and priorities'. Available at: www.rcpsych.ac.uk/docs/default-source/improving-care/better-mh-policy/policy/rcpsych---improving-mental-health-services-in-systems-of-integrated-and-accountable-care-final.pdf (Accessed: 9 March 2023).

Samaritans. (2017) 'Dying from inequality: Socioeconomic disadvantage and suicidal behaviour'. Available at: https://media.samaritans.org/documents/Samaritans_Dying_from_inequality_report_-_summary.pdf (Accessed 24 January 2023).

Sareen, J., Erickson, J., Medved, M.I., Asmundson, G.J., Enns, M.W., Stein, M., Leslie, W., Doupe, M. and Logsetty, S. (2013) 'Risk factors for post-injury mental health problems', *Depression and Anxiety*, 30(4), pp. 321–327.

Schneider, F., Erhart, M., Hewer, W., Loeffler, L.A. and Jacobi, F. (2019) 'Mortality and medical comorbidity in the severely mentally ill: a German registry study', *Deutsches Ärzteblatt International*, 116(23–24), pp. 405–411.

Scott, R., Aboud, A. and Smith, T. (2022) 'Using the stress–vulnerability model to better understand suicide in prison populations', *Psychiatry, Psychology and Law*, online ahead-of-print.

Scott, A. J., Webb, T. L., Martyn-St James, M., Rowse, G. and Weich, S. (2021) 'Improving sleep quality leads to better mental health: A meta-analysis of randomised controlled trials', *Sleep Medicine Reviews*, 60, pp. 1–9.

Ser, G., Robertson, A. and Sheikh, A. (2014) 'A qualitative exploration of workarounds related to the implementation of national electronic health records in early adopter mental health hospitals', *PloS ONE*, 9(1), pp. 1–9.

Sharp, P., Bottorff, J. L., Rice, S., Oliffe, J. L., Schulenkorf, N., Impellizzeri, F. and Caperchione, C. M. (2022) '"People say men don't talk, well that's bullshit": A focus group study exploring challenges and opportunities for men's mental health promotion', *PLoS One*, 17(1), pp. 1–17.

Simpson, A., Hannigan, B., Coffey, M., Jones, A., Barlow, S., Cohen, R., Všetečková, J. and Faulkner, A. (2016) 'Cross-national comparative mixed-methods case study of recovery-focused mental health care planning and co-ordination: Collaborative Care Planning Project (COCAPP)', *Health Services and Delivery Research*, 4(5), pp. 1–190.

Smuts, J. (1926) *Holism and Evolution*. London: MacMillian and Co.

Stiawa, M., Müller-Stierlin, A., Staiger, T., Killan, R., Becker, T., Günder, H., Beschoner, P., Grinschgl, A., Frasch, K., Schmauß, M., Panzirsch, M., Mayer, L., Sittenbuger, E. and Krumm, S. (2020) 'Mental health professionals view about the impact of male gender for the treatment of men with depression – a qualitative study', *BMC Psychiatry*, 20(276), pp. 1–13.

Sullivan, L.E., Fiellin, D.A. and O'Connor, P.G. (2005) 'The prevalence and impact of alcohol problems in major depression: a systematic review', *The American Journal of Medicine*, 118(4), pp. 330–341.

Thornton, L. (2019) 'A brief history and overview of holistic nursing', *Integrative Medicine: A Clinician's Journal*, 18(4), pp. 32–33.

Tol, W.A., Bastin, P., Jordans, M.J., Minas, H., Souza, R., Weissbecker, I. and Van Ommeren, M. (2013) 'Mental Health and Psychosocial Support in Humanitarian Settings', in V. Patel, H. Minas, A. Cohen and M. Prince (Eds) *Global Mental Health: Principles and Practice*. Oxford: Oxford University Press, pp. 384–389.

Treede, R.D. (2018) 'The International Association for the Study of Pain definition of pain: as valid in 2018 as in 1979, but in need of regularly updated footnotes', *Pain Reports*, 3(2), pp. 1–2.

United Nations. (2015) 'The 17 goals: Sustainable development'. Available at: https://sdgs.un.org/goals (Accessed: 12 April 2023).

Wilding, J. (2014) 'The importance of weight management in type 2 diabetes mellitus', *International Journal of Clinical Practice*, 68(6), pp. 682–691.

Williamson, V., Diehle, J., Dunn, R., Jones, N. and Greenberg, N. (2019) 'The impact of military service on health and well-being', *Occupational Medicine*, 69(1), pp. 64–70.

Workforce Institute. (2023) 'The impact of work on mental health'. Available at: https://workforceinstitute.org/the-impact-of-work-on-mental-health/#:~:text=A%20new%20global%20study%20from,spouse%20or%20partner%20(69%25) (Accessed: 12 April 2023).

World Health Organization (2020) 'Mental health atlas'. Available at: www.who.int/publications/i/item/9789240036703 (Accessed: 12 April 2023).

World Health Organization (2021) 'Comprehensive mental health action plan'. Available at: www.who.int/publications/i/item/9789240031029 (Accessed: 12 April 2023).

World Health Organization. (2022) 'World mental health report: Transforming mental health for all executive summary'. Available at: www.who.int/publications/i/item/9789240050860 (Accessed: 12 April 2023).

Zubin, J. and Spring, B. (1977) 'Vulnerability: A new view of schizophrenia', *Journal of Abnormal Psychology*, 86(2), pp. 103–126.

7 Global Health Pillar

Joel Faronbi, Faye Doris, Susan Clompus, and Jasmine Hesslegrave

Introduction

Health and social care provision varies from one country, region, and geographical location to another and is impacted by complex socio-demographic and economic factors (Robertson, Gregory, and Jabbal, 2014). Different efforts and approaches to address health, at the international level, brought about the concept of global health. Global health refers to responses to health challenges and responses and efforts to improve health and achieve equity/reduce and eradicate disparities, that are not limited to a particular geographical location, and which go beyond the capacity of a single country to manage (Beaglehole and Bonita, 2010). As part of global health challenges, nurses need to update their knowledge and skills to be equipped to work in new and emerging transnational contexts (Bradbury-Jones and Clark, 2017).

This chapter discusses health as a global phenomenon and nurses' responses towards addressing health issues that transcend national borders (McMichael and Butler, 2006). The chapter starts with a scenario about the activities of a migrant nurse, Titi, who observed similarities and differences in the role as a community health nurse in her home country, Nigeria, as compared with the United Kingdom (UK). The chapter explores the impact of current and future global health challenges which impact health and social care including care workforce shortages and migration, global disease threats such as pandemics, common health challenges including pollution and the climate crisis. We conclude with a reflection on sustainable nursing practice sensitive to diverse cultural contexts.

Scenario

Titi is a registered nurse from Nigeria who migrated to the UK as she wished to broaden her career and continue to develop professionally. She has left her husband and two children back in Nigeria but hopes that they will be able to join her sometime in the future. Her elderly mother in Nigeria, who earns some money from buying and selling items, helps with the care of the children.

On arrival in the UK, Titi worked in a nursing home in the social care sector, while working towards her registration as a nurse in the UK. Following registration with the UK Nursing and

DOI: 10.4324/9781003390565-7

Midwifery Council (NMC), she took up a position as a registered nurse in an infection control team in a local National Health Service (NHS) hospital.

Titi had extensive experience as a nurse in a range of global health conditions such as malaria, tuberculosis, measles, and HIV/AIDS, prior to her arrival in the UK. She also worked as a community health nurse, where she participated in community assessment and interventions for local health related conditions. Titi also had some exposure to international organisations such as the United Nations (UN) International Children's Emergency Fund (UNICEF) and the World Health Organization (WHO). Working with these organisations, Titi participated in programmes such as the national programme on immunisation, a national water, sanitation and hygiene programme, and other efforts by non-governmental organisations (NGOs) to eradicate communicable and non-communicable diseases and malnutrition in populations. Titi also participated in training and facilitated some community health programmes, including local staff training in the integrated management of childhood illness. She hopes that she will be able to share this knowledge and experience through contributing to patient care, education, and research in the UK.

Titi is committed to developing her knowledge further and recently read about the emergence and re-emergence of new and old infectious diseases respectfully, and wondered why this is so. She is ambitious to complete an infectious diseases course and to specialise in this field of care. She learns of the experiences of UK nurses during the COVID-19 pandemic and compares this to her own experience during the COVID-19 pandemic in Nigeria.

Titi is aware that staff nurses in the UK have some knowledge of the climate crisis and its links to global health and would like to do some teaching in this area. She is aware that scientists are expecting an increased prevalence of malaria and other tropically related conditions in the UK, due to rising temperatures and migration of mosquitoes through air travel.

Global Health

Global health refers to health issues affecting most countries. It is a relatively new concept replacing the previous focus on tropical medicine and international health that were linked to the history of colonialism and developmental assistance, among the European colonies (Birn, Pillay, and Holtz, 2017; Holst, 2020; Worboys, 2000). In addition, the focus on global and international health has historically been used to describe health issues in lower income countries from the biased perspective of higher income countries.

The concept of 'global health' came into existence within the past 20 years. The concept has been expanded to incorporate how countries relate with one another on health matters and how their relationship affects the planet's health (Bradbury-Jones and Clark, 2017). It has been adopted by many governments and organisations as a key policy theme. As nurses, we need to consider the impact of factors that affect health in other places that may indirectly impact our health and that of our family and the communities we serve. For example, the catchphrase 'Think globally, act locally!' in terms of the response to COVID-19 resonates this with premise (Hoff, 2015, p. 28). As nurses, we are obliged to understand the world in its broader context and base decision-making on an expanded understanding of ourselves, the patients we assist, and our circumstances.

Global health reflects the realities of globalisation, migration, increased movement of persons and goods and associated risk of infectious and non-infectious conditions (De Haas, 2011). Global health is also concerned with efforts designed to protect the entire global community, both poor and rich, against threats to health and with delivering essential and cost-effective public health and clinical services to the world's population (De Haas, 2011). This is with the view that no country can ensure the health of its population in isolation from the rest of the world (De Cock et al., 2013).

In the past, the discussion on global and international health was mainly centred on infectious diseases such as influenza, tuberculosis, yellow fever, and cholera because of their prevalence among low-and middle-income nations. This assertion has been expanded because communicable and non-communicable diseases ravage lives in different countries, irrespective of their location or economic status.

Although common, global health is difficult to define because it includes public health, tropical health, and global health governance. Koplan et al. (2009) stated that global health has areas of overlap with the more established public health and international health disciplines. Often global health is used interchangeably with 'international health', but conceptualising it this way may limit global health to the disparity in health between low- and high-income nations.

Global health can thus be defined as a broad area of study, research, and practice that prioritises improving health and achieving equity in health for all people worldwide (Koplan et al., 2009), ensuring health-promoting and sustainable sociocultural, political, and economic systems (Jones and Sherwood, 2014). Global health emphasises transnational health issues, determinants, and solutions, is multidisciplinary in nature, extends beyond health sciences, promotes interdisciplinary collaborations and is a synthesis of population-based prevention with individual and holistic clinical care (Koplan et al., 2009). Global health also implies planetary health, which equals human, animal, environmental and ecosystem health (Kahn et al., 2014).

Recently, the discussions on global health have been expanded to include long-term conditions and obesity, climate change, urbanisation, health equity, social injustice, and income disparities linked to health across nations. It also encompasses political discussions and controversies around science, governance, ethics, and health policy frameworks (World Health Organization, 2013a, 2013b).

Global health is intrinsically linked to political instability. It has been documented that the health system, in some countries, is weakened due to political instability. A classic example could be seen in the Russia and Venezuela, where the political instability in both countries triggered the outbreak of malaria, tuberculosis, and diphtheria (Claborn, 2018).

These are some features distinguishing global health from the more restrictive field of international health. For instance, one definition of global health has been described as the range of health issues influenced by factors that extend beyond state borders, including preparedness for pandemic influenza and emerging infections and climate change (Department of Health, 2011). Global health focuses on issues that directly or indirectly affect health that transcends national boundaries, while international health focuses on health issues of countries other than one's own, especially those of low-income and middle-income. In addition, global health often requires global cooperation, while international health usually requires binational cooperation (Koplan et al., 2009). Global health provides interaction among nations through foreign policy, thereby achieving national and global security, creating economic wealth, supporting development in low-income countries, and promoting human dignity through the protection of human rights and the delivery of humanitarian assistance (United Nations General Assembly, 2015). Amorim-Maia et al. (2022) argued that focusing on inequities and social justice is key to understanding the difference between international and global health. Similarly, Claborn (2018) further argued that the perspective of international health from the safe harbour of the 'developed' world is myopic and insufficient.

History and Background to International Global Health Events and Declarations

In 1851, the first international discussion on public health took place in Paris in response to an ongoing cholera epidemic. The meeting was tagged as the first international sanitary conference focusing on the international community's appropriate response to public health emergencies. The forum allowed international cooperation and discussion on pressing health issues. Later, in the late 19th century and early 20th centuries, sanitary conferences were convened on an ad hoc basis until the birth of the World Health Organization on 7 April 1948 (Birn, Pillay, and Holtz, 2017). Throughout its history, the WHO has been the key driver of major global health initiatives, including eradicating smallpox and the creation of the Framework Convention on Tobacco Control. WHO guidelines and statistics are used to inform decision-making in both high-income and low- and middle-income countries.

In 1978, the first-ever international conference on primary care, convened by the WHO and UN Children's Fund (UNICEF), took place in Almaty in Kazakhstan, leading to the Declaration of Alma-Ata which birthed a landmark moment in the history of global health (World Health Organization, 1978). It endorsed the primary care approach to improving health, emphasising the need to tackle health's social, political, and economic determinants. It also endorsed a vision of health for all by the year 2000 and health was linked with global security.

The eight Millennium Development Goals (MDGs) – which range from halving extreme poverty rates to halting the spread of HIV/AIDS and providing universal primary education, all by the target date of 2015 – formed a blueprint agreed by the UN member states. The failure to meet the earlier target bore the Rio+20, also known as the Sustainable development UN conference, in 2012.

The Sustainable Development Goals (SDGs) provide a call to action for all global countries, irrespective of their wealth status, to promote prosperity while securing the environment. They recognise that to end poverty, other strategies must exist, including education, health, social protection, and job opportunities required for economic sustainability and addressing a range of social needs, while also tackling climate change and environmental protection. Building on the progress of the MDG, they recognised the need to set more objectives with achievable targets for each of the goals. The Sustainable Development Goals (SDGs) are world-changing objectives requiring cooperation among governments, international organisations, world leaders, and individuals (Lim et al., 2016; Manyazewal, 2017). One of the slogans for the SDG is 'Change starts with me' (United Nations, 2016). It is believed that every human is part of the solution. Fortunately, there are some easy things we can adopt to make a difference.

For effective change in the health sector, nurses must be proactive. For our activities to count, nurses must be actively involved in global health initiatives, adopting the phrase

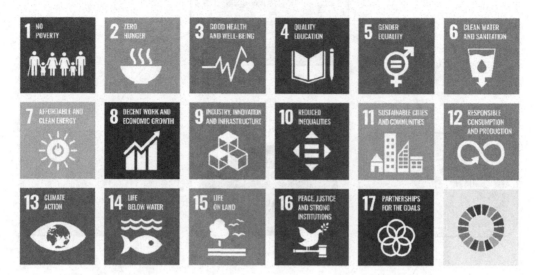

Figure 7.1 Sustainable Development Goals

Source: www.un.org/sustainabledevelopment/

'thinking globally and acting locally' (Hoff, 2015, p. 28) by adopting a mindset that seeks to understand the structural and political conditions that sustain armed conflict, poverty, inequality, inaction on environmental pollution, and poorer health and well-being of vulnerable populations (Salvage and White, 2020). For a change to be meaningful, it must have an evidence base (Titler, 2008). Implementing evidence-based change must also require political and ethical awareness alongside action, and Figure 7.1 illustrates the wide-ranging goals involved with promoting a sustainable world from stopping poverty, inequalities, and climate change.

A Model of Global Health

A model of global health is presented with this discussion. The model stipulates that global health results from interaction among the model's core components, including common health challenges, migration, global disease threats, and climate change. Each of the variables interacts with one another, resulting in what is known as global health. Using the example of malaria, the global health model suggests that better protection for a human population might be gained by addressing the underlying economic and social inequities that allow disease transmission or the most serious disease manifestations to occur. Those underlying inequities might lead to inadequate housing that lacks window screens and doors, insufficient access to health care, lack of appropriate education, or nutritional deficiencies that perpetuate severe manifestations of the disease. A detailed discussion on each of the concepts in the model will be provided to aid an in-depth understanding of the chapter.

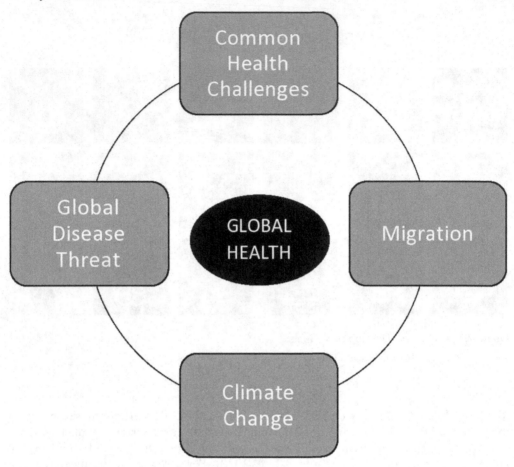

Figure 7.2 Global health model

Migration and Care Workforce Shortages

An increased number of people are migrating from the global south to the global north because of conflict and other political, demographic, socio-economic and environmental situations (Castelli, 2018; Li, Nie, and Li, 2014). The recruitment of nurses, doctors and other health and social care workers from the south to the north, to meet the staffing crisis in organisations such as the NHS in the UK, is commonplace and contentious (Waitzman, 2022). According to NHS Digital, as of June 2022, 4% (9,400) of nurses in NHS employment are of African nationality and 5,537 are Nigerian (Baker, 2022). With the current acute shortage and massive drive for recruitment, this figure is likely to have increased. This recruitment is a global trend seen across Europe, North America, and Australasia as healthcare organisations strive to meet their staffing crisis. It leaves us with a challenge and questioning of this practice on an ethical and professional basis. Who does it benefit? Who is harmed? and what does it offer?

Benefits to the recruiting countries include increased staff, something that Titi would contribute to. It may also be argued that Titi would acquire additional professional experience, skills, and knowledge. There is a loss to the healthcare system that Titi has left as Titi made a valuable contribution to Nigerian health care. This has provoked many conversations around what is right and what is wrong, meriting the continuing ethical and professional debates about this at local, national, and international levels. Through such debate, offers learning and the sharing of experiences with opportunity to develop understanding of the WHO principles (Aluttis, Bishaw and Frank, 2014).

Globally, there is an impact of increased nurses' migration from the source countries to the recipient countries (Li, Nie, and Li, 2014). This impact is felt in both countries. Some source countries may be left with a collapsing health system, while the recipient countries use these opportunities to fill vacancies. This global phenomenon stems from historical, economic, social, and political factors. The impact of migration has a significant effect on individual and national levels, with a positive and negative impact on the source country (Li, Nie, and Li, 2014). A significant effect is a remittance received from the host countries to foreign countries, often used to boost the economy of the source countries. The migrant is, however, also seen as contributing to the local economy through remittances and the reduction of unemployment (Lorenzo et al., 2007). In addition, migration provides an opportunity for knowledge enhancement for those nurses who could return to their home countries after acquiring some grasp of health technologies used abroad.

Migration also has the potential to impact the economy of a nation. The potential for migrants and diasporas to positively impact development in their countries of origin, mainly through their remittances, has been argued (Gelb et al., 2021). The UN also states that leveraging remittances for development is vital for achieving the SDGs and includes remittances under SDG 10, Reducing inequality within and among countries (Gelb et al., 2021). Remittance enables migrants and diasporas to fully contribute to sustainable development in all countries (Gelb et al., 2021). The migrant was, however, also seen as contributing to the local economy through remittances and the reduction of unemployment (Lorenzo et al., 2007).

According to World Bank 2005 report, Pakistan, after India, is one of the second largest countries among the recipients of remittances in South Asian Countries, which is received mainly by the families left behind (Ariadi et al., 2019; World Bank, 2005). It represents key factors which help avoid the adverse effects of macroeconomic shocks, having countercyclical character (Đukić and Bodroža, 2022; Chami, Hakura and Montiel, 2009). Stable remittance inflows significantly contributed to the stability of the exchange rate, even putting pressure to appreciate (increases in the value of a capital asset over time) (Đukić and Bodroža, 2022; Chami, Hakura and Montiel, 2009). However, there are social and economic repercussion for unmanaged migration, economic gains are likely to be wiped out by family, psychological, and social losses. Some may be seen in Titi's family as she has left her husband and children behind thus, creating a social loss.

In other words, migration also impacts negatively. One such impact is the depletion of skilled workers. A classic example is seen in the Philippines, where a shortage of highly skilled nurses has created severe problems for the Philippines health system, including the closure of many hospitals (Lorenzo et al., 2007; Kingma, 2018). Migration was perceived to negatively impact nursing in the Philippines by depleting the pool of skilled and experienced health workers, thus compromising the quality of care in the health care system. One concern among health services managers is that the loss of more senior nurses requires continual investment in training staff replacements and negatively affects the quality of care. Similarly, the cost of human resources increases given that mass migration results in a depleted workforce (Lorenzo et al., 2007).

Studies suggest that parental migration can contribute to reduced mental health among left-behind family members; children may be more vulnerable to mental health conditions such as depression, emotional disturbance, anxiety and fear, and lower self-esteem (Kahn et al., 2014; Adumitroaie and Dafinoiu, 2013). It is also associated with poorer physical and mental health outcomes of ageing parents (Thapa et al., 2018; Ariadi, Saud, and Ashfaq, 2019). Migration has been shown to lead to the absence of parental care and supervision, and low family support was related to mental disorders (Shen et al., 2015). In another example, the left-behind children in Sri Lanka had a higher prevalence of mental health problems and were more likely to have conflicts with peers and teachers, have more anxiety, lower self-esteem, higher suicidal behaviour, and higher substance abuse than children living with their parents (Wang et al., 2011; Shen et al., 2015; Valtolina and Colombo, 2012).

There is, then, evidence that migration contributes negatively to the health of the left behind children. This might be observed in some nurses such as Titi, leaving her infants supported by relatives, increasing the risk of some adverse consequences if caregivers are not able to provide the same level of support as the parent(s). It is important to add the voice of the International Council of Nurses (ICN) to this discussion which states that 'Any international recruitment should adhere to WHO's global code of practice on international recruitment and follow ICN's guidance concerning nurses' welfare and employment rights, and the requirements of the countries that are supplying nurses to the rest of the world' (International Council of Nurses, 2021).

Global Disease Threats

The movement of people creates exposure to new pathogens and risk behaviours. The discovery of the 'New World' and the Americas by early European settlers exposed local populations to the previously unknown smallpox pathogen. Historically, Europeans exposed indigenous peoples to smallpox and measles with deadly consequences, while Europeans died from malaria and yellow fever, which were predominant in tropical overseas countries. Many white settlers/workers/soldiers and their dependents died in Africa and India from these infectious diseases (Dumett, 1968; MacLeod and Lewis, 2022). So, the need to control and study tropical diseases became imperative as infections limited the potential for the economic exploitation of newly acquired territories. As a result, new institutions for the study of tropical medicine were established (Claborn, 2018; Behbehani, 1983; Hirsch and Martin, 2022). Today, in the era of air travel, pathogens have the potential to spread rapidly around the world, and the importance of institutions of tropical health remains undiminished. Human migration has been the pathway for disseminating infectious diseases and will continue to shape the pattern of the spread of infections in geographic areas and populations (Wilson, 1995; Church, 2004); Some of these diseases include plagues and dengue fever, Smallpox (Wilson, 1995), Ebola (Otu et al., 2018), respiratory virus pathogens (Ikonen et al., 2018), COVID-19 (Sharma, 2020), and many others. Titi's employment in the infection control team is well placed as she hopes to pursue an infection control course and to become a specialist nurse in this field.

Common Health Problems

Common health problems (CHPs) include conditions such as pain, fatigue, and depression which are prevalent among the general population (Barnes et al., 2008). CHPs are not necessarily interpreted as pathological or disabling, but they can be chronic with distressing complaints (Barnes et al., 2008). The individual may present an array of subjective complaints, sometimes difficult to correlate with pathological reports (Buck et al., 2010). They have a high prevalence in the general population and are typically mild and self-limiting (Buck et al., 2010). They can become chronic and distressing, resulting in long-term sickness and absence from work. They may be associated with poor outcomes, isolation, increased risks of poverty, and physical and mental health problems (Henderson et al., 2011). They are often cited as reasons for seeking medical advice, sickness absence, and long-term incapacity for work (Buck et al., 2010). CHPs can be caused or associated with many factors including climate change and climate crisis. Among Nigerians, the most prevalent health conditions are joint pain, general body pains, and blurring of vision, febrile illness, musculoskeletal-related disorders (especially osteoarthritis), cardiovascular problems (especially hypertension), and respiratory problems (cough and catarrh) (Abegunde and Owoaje, 2013; Faronbi, Ajadi and Gobbens, 2020).

The Climate Crisis and Global Health

The earth is our only support system, there is no planet B. The current climate crisis poses perilous consequences for human life and the health effect of climate change has been well documented (Lipp, Huq and Colwell, 2002; McMichael, Woodruff and Hales, 2006; Majra and Gur, 2009). These include natural and environmental disasters, such as floods, storms, and cyclones, prevalence of vector-borne diseases, injuries, and deaths due to extreme weather conditions and others. This impact on all the components of health including mental health is likely to be substantial (McMichael and Butler, 2006; Padhy et al., 2015). Children and the older adults are particularly vulnerable to the health impacts of climate change as their immune systems are inefficient/ineffective/incompetent, leaving them more susceptible to disease and environmental pollutants. The damage done in early childhood lasts a lifetime. The impacts of climate crisis and global health will be further discussed under the following subsections: extreme weather events, the impact of water availability, increased spread of diseases, mass displacement, poverty and financial instability, and the threat of new diseases.

Extreme Weather

According to the Lancet countdown report 2021, people suffer due to extreme weather events such as droughts, storms, ocean warming, floods, fires and increases in extreme weather events such as heat waves, and sea level rise (Beggs et al., 2022). Consider the recent case of Pakistan, which caused flooding the size of the UK. Heatwaves can cause heat stress and impacts on patients with heart failure for example. Storms and floods cause injuries, loss of life, livelihoods, the potential hospital shut down, and disease outbreaks. These weather events impact on people's mental health through stress and trauma. Wildfires also dramatically worsen air pollution in some areas. Extreme weather and soil degradation also impact food production and water availability, leading to increased risks of health impacts through starvation, dehydration, and malnutrition. Moreover, global heating reduces crop yields and shrinks nutrients in cereal crops impacting malnutrition (Hanjra and Qureshi, 2010).

Increased Spread of Diseases

Higher temperatures help bacteria that cause deadly diarrhoea (and wound infections) to thrive, leading to the increased spread of infectious diseases such as cholera. Hotter temperatures increase the frequency mosquitoes feed off humans, while increased rainfall creates more stagnant water sources for these deadly insects to breed. Mosquitoes are considered one of the most dangerous species on the planet due to their ability to spread many deadly diseases such as Zika virus, West Nile virus, chikungunya virus infections, dengue fever and malaria (Anoopkumar and Aneesh, 2022). A growing number of scientists are concerned that global warming could lead to an explosive growth of mosquito-borne diseases worldwide, a problem that will be exacerbated by mosquitoes becoming increasingly resistant to insecticides. Other tropical diseases are beginning to be seen in uncommon parts of the world, for example, chikungunya fever, Zika, encephalitis and canine heartworm, some of which have been found in isolated parts of southern England (El-Sayed and Kamel, 2020). Zika virus, which causes congenital disabilities, has been found in France and could spread to the UK soon (Cugola, Fernandes and Russo, 2016).

Malaria and dengue are now in Europe and the UK (Bayliss, 2017). In addition, hotter temperatures mean resistance to some antibiotics (Collignon et al., 2018). Nigeria bears 25% of the global malaria burden (Tola et al., 2020), and malaria is ranked as the number one cause of morbidity and mortality in both adults and children (World Health Organization, 2008). The current global climate crisis (increased rainfall, temperature, and relative humidity) is favourable for mosquito abundance and its associated malaria morbidity (Jonathan et al., 2018; Adeola et al., 2017). Similarly, long-distance migration of some species of *Anopheles* mosquito may also be implicated in the spread of diseases (Huestis et al., 2019; Dao et al., 2014).

Other threats also include overfishing and mercury pollution in European waters (Zhang et al., 2022); soil degradation; damage to potatoes, cauliflowers, and cabbages resulting in reductions in food supplies (Saeed et al., 2023); and shrink in the level of nutrients in crops leading to malnutrition (Agostoni et al., 2023).

Health Threats from Air Pollution

Air pollutants are produced through the uncontrolled burning of fossil fuels. Exposure to air pollutants has been linked to an increased risk of premature mortality, respiratory disorders, cardiovascular diseases (CVD) and mental disorders (Gu et al., 2020), and damage to the nervous system (Shabani, 2021). There is also a danger of industrial accidents, associated with wide spread of a toxic fog which can be fatal to the populations of the surrounding areas (Manisalidis et al., 2020). Air pollution has raised the morbidity and mortality in some countries. For example, in China, lung cancer mortality has been associated with fine particles found in air pollution (Kan, Chen, and Tong, 2012). Similarly, in India, Chronic obstructive respiratory disease, lung cancer, and acute lower respiratory disease were observed in women and young children under 5 years of age, respectively (Dherani et al., 2008). Also, in Nigeria, a lot of industrial activities such as mining, construction and factories cause air pollution and resultant health consequences seen on daily basis (Ajibola et al., 2020). Of immense importance is the oil-generated environmental pollution and degradation occurring in the Niger Delta region of the country (Ukaogo et al., 2020; Edna, Ateboh, and Raimi, 2018). The consequence of air pollution has also been seen in the death of an asthmatic child in London, UK from exhaust fumes (Laville, 2020).

Threat of New Diseases

There is a potential risk of new diseases, for example, Spanish flu, buried in the permafrost (Charlier et al., 2017) or the risk of diseases jumping from animal to human origin due to the degradation of natural habitats (Keesing et al., 2010). For example, deforestation in Malaysia and Singapore caused fruit bats carrying the Nipah virus to move from the forest to fruit plantations, passing the virus onto pigs and then transmitting it to humans (Ma et al., 2009). It also includes the spread of crop pests and diseases to new parts of the world, for example, the *Xylella* bacterium (Pavlović et al., 2022), and 'wheat blast' (Marchioro et al., 2023), alongside other antibiotic resistance diseases (Bebber et al., 2014). One of the emerging diseases in Nigeria is human monkeypox. The 2022 outbreak presented with an unusual pattern and have no epidemiological connection with countries that previously reported human monkeypox (Ilic et al., 2022).

Impact of Water Availability

According to the UN World Water Development Report in 2018, 3.6 billion people (nearly half the global population) live in water-scarce areas for at least one month per year. This situation is exacerbated by hotter, drier conditions and more frequent and extreme droughts. In 2017 a drought in East Africa displaced 800,000 people in Somalia (Hujale, 2022). In 2018 an intense drought in Cape Town led to severe water restrictions being put in place, and the city came to within days of turning off its water supply. Day Zero is known when a city's taps dry out, and people must stand in line to collect a daily water quota (Waxa, 2020). The melting of glaciers has impacted water availability. Today, around 1.9 billion people live in catchment areas downstream of glaciated mountain ranges and depend on glaciers for clean water. However, these glaciers are rapidly melting (Dasgupta et al., 2009). Nigeria is situated in West Africa and the region has been regarded as one of the most susceptible regions to climate change, any tilt toward dryness in the future climate may deteriorate the risk of severe drought to the area. Drought has been directly or indirectly linked to water scarcity as well as many other environmental problems (Ogunrinde et al., 2022).

Mass Displacement, Poverty, and Financial Instability

Climate change has already led to global inequality. Extreme weather can displace people from their countries and homes. Climate change and overuse of natural resources are among the highest risk to security, with an impact far higher than weapons of mass destruction (Titus et al., 2023). Extreme weather events, made more likely by climate change, already cause substantial financial losses and threaten to make our world systemically uninsurable (Philipsborn et al., 2021). Lack of climate action, biodiversity loss and extreme weather is one of the biggest threats to the global economy resulting in mass displacement, poverty, social instability, and conflict around resources by 2050 or the end of the century (United Nations, 2020). In Nigeria, large-scale involuntary internal displacement caused by armed conflicts such as the terrorist activities by members of the Boko Haram insurgency group (Faronbi et al., 2019) and flooding natural disasters are reported to cause the deaths of more than 600 people with 1.4 million people displaced, and thousands of hectares of submerged farmland (Olagunju et al., 2021).

Sustainable Nursing Practice

The COVID-19 pandemic reinforced the relationship between global health and healthcare systems worldwide. It has been recognised that healthcare systems' carbon emissions negatively impact the health of local and global populations (Lenzen et al., 2020; NHS England, 2022). In England, the I (2008) set national targets for reducing carbon emissions. The target was set in recognition of the estimated number of lives that could be saved per year from a net zero healthcare system (NHS England, 2022). The current analysis predicts that 5,770 lives could be saved a year by reducing air pollution in the UK alone (NHS England, 2022). Therefore, a target was set up, and if achieved could see improvements in health universally. In an attempt to reduce the NHS's carbon footprint by 80% by 2040, NHS England has recognised that a priority should be to reduce air pollution. If this target is to be achieved, several concerted efforts must be put in place to reduce air pollution; this includes incorporating green spaces into healthcare settings, engineering solutions, and appropriate use of single-use products.

Reducing air pollution can be done by incorporating green spaces into healthcare settings. Green environments have known benefits for physical and mental health (Marques da Costa and Kállay, 2020). Incorporating green environments will increase the number of species that remove carbon emissions from local environments, reducing air pollution and benefiting the local population's health (Browning, Rigolon, and McAnirlin, 2022).

In addition to green spaces, engineering solutions can be utilised to develop infrastructure to ensure estate facilities are limiting their carbon emissions. Engineering solutions which may initially cost to ensure efficient energy systems are installed will eventually save an approximated £14.3 million per year in the UK alone. Energy monitoring, insulation, heat distribution and renewable energy demonstrate a commitment to reducing carbon emissions (NHS England, 2022).

Another effort to reduce carbon footprint is the appropriate use of single-use products. During COVID-19, the health services understandably used enormous amounts of personal protection equipment (PPE) to maintain patient care and to reduce transmission of the disease. Concerns about the impact this is having on environmental and public health can be addressed at the grassroot level by healthcare leaders to raise educational awareness of when PPE should be used to reduce the unnecessary use of single-use plastics within healthcare (Shepherd, 2019).

Conclusion

This chapter provides a discussion of health on the global scene, scaffolded around a scenario about a person called Titi who emigrated to England to qualify as a nurse. Focus was on transnational and transborder health issues and promoting multidisciplinary and interdisciplinary collaborations for the synthesis of population-based intervention. The chapter provided historical background to global health and linked this to some international global health events and declarations; notable is the first international discussion on public health which took place in Paris in response to the cholera epidemic and the birth of the World Health Organization in 1948. Further examined, was global health using a uniquely designed model to elaborate on the core components of global health, including common health challenges, migration, global disease threats, and climate change.

The scenario relating to Titi, prompts reflection on the global healthcare workforce shortages which nurses' decisions to migrate from, for example, the global south to the north. The attendant consequences on the source and recipient countries, including knowledge enhancement and contributing to the local economy mainly through their remittances, were explored. Negative impacts of migration, including depletion of skilled workers and reduced physical and mental health, were also discussed in the light of ICN recommendations relating to ethical and equitable recruitment of international health workers. Global disease threats, associated with migration, were also considered as were the grave consequences of human activities on the planet contributing to the climate crisis. Health implications arising from extreme weather conditions, increased disease prevalence, air pollution, the emergence of new diseases, food and water shortage were introduced. This is alongside mass displacement, poverty, and financial instability. In addition, several concerted efforts to reduce air pollution, such as green spaces in healthcare settings, engineering solutions, and appropriate use of single-use products, were presented. Nurses have a critical role to play in the advancement of global health through education, practice, and research, and it is the chapter develops understanding of global health issues, and sparks interest and debate about considering health from a global perspective.

Takeaways for Student Nurses

- Nurses are the largest cadre of healthcare workers and are largely responsible for patient care worldwide, often referred to as the 'backbone of healthcare systems'. Nurses are on the frontline of detecting, treating, and preventing infectious diseases in many settings.
- The chapter illustrates that nurse education and practice extend beyond the local, regional, or national, therefore, student nurses require to build understanding about nursing care practices that has global health at its heart.
- Nurses have responsibilities to improve the health and wellbeing of all the world's citizens. Student nurses should be prepared to deliver culturally sensitive care touched upon in the patient involvement chapter to patients, families, and communities.
- Nurse education should be comprehensive to encompass the biopsychosocial determinants of health and students should learn how they could apply this beyond the primary, secondary, and tertiary care systems.
- Student nurses should work within the multi-professional team to promote healthy environments and sustainable development and with interpersonal abilities to develop local and global partnerships.

Takeaways for Educators/Practitioners

- Globalisation brings about emerging and remerging health conditions; therefore, nurses must respond proactively to global health challenges and understand the effects of globalisation on health worldwide.
- Nurses must assume leadership roles locally and globally to advocate for the wellbeing of individuals, families and communities and the planet, as well as engaging in critical thinking through wide reading and debate regarding social, economic, and health issues integrated into a global event.
- We must seek knowledge on political, economic, and social matters associated with the scarcity of financial and technological resources and use our broad nursing knowledge to influence change.
- Nurses must collaborate with other professionals to perform within the perspective of a healthy environment and sustainable development. This is adopting interpersonal abilities to develop local and global partnerships with awareness and mitigation of environmental impacts such as carbon emissions.
- The current global mass migration of nurses calls for advocating responsible recruitment to allow for ethical and equitable distribution of human resources for health services worldwide.

References

Abegunde, K. and Owoaje, E. (2013). 'Health problems and associated risk factors in selected urban and rural elderly population groups of south-west Nigeria', *Annals of African Medicine*, 12, pp. 90–97.

Adeola, A. M., Botai, J. O., Rautenbach, H., Adisa, O. M., Ncongwane, K. P., Botai, C. M. and Adebayo-Ojo, T. C. (2017) 'Climatic variables and malaria morbidity in mutual local municipality, south Africa: A 19-year data analysis', *International Journal of Environmental Research and Public Health*, 14, pp. 1360–1375.

Adumitroaie, E. and Dafinoiu, I. (2013). 'Perception of parental rejection in children left behind by migrant parents', *Revista de cercetare si interventie sociala*, 42, pp. 191–203.

Agostoni, C., Baglioni, M., La Vecchia, A., Molari, G. and Berti, C. (2023) 'Interlinkages between climate change and food systems: The impact on child malnutrition—narrative review', *Nutrients*, 15(2), p. 1–15.

Ajibola, A. F., Raimi, M. O., Steve-Awogbami, O. C., Adeniji, A. O. and Adekunle, A. P. (2020). 'Policy responses to addressing the issues of environmental health impacts of charcoal factory in Nigeria: Necessity today; essentiality tomorrow', *Communication, Society and Media*, 3(3), pp. 2576–5388.

Aluttis, C., Bishaw, T. and Frank, M. W. (2014) 'The workforce for health in a globalized context–global shortages and international migration', *Global Health Action*, 7(23611) pp. 1–7.

Amorim-Maia, A.T., Anguelovski, I., Chu, E. and Connolly, J., (2022) 'Intersectional climate justice: A conceptual pathway for bridging adaptation planning, transformative action, and social equity', *Urban Climate*, 41, pp. 1–18.

Anoopkumar, A.N. and Aneesh, E.M. (2022) 'A critical assessment of mosquito control and the influence of climate change on mosquito-borne disease epidemics', *Environment, Development and Sustainability*, 24(6), pp. 8900–8929.

Ariadi, S., Saud, M. and Ashfaq, A. (2019) 'Analyzing the effect of remittance transfer on socio-economic well-being of left-behind parents: A study of Pakistan and Azad Jammu and Kashmir (ajk)', *Journal of International Migration and Integration*, 20, pp. 809–821.

Baker, C. (2022) 'Nationality of NHS staff in England'. Available at: https://researchbriefings.files.parliament.uk/documents/CBP-7783/CBP-7783.pdf (Accessed: 17 April 2023).

Baylis, M. (2017) 'Potential impact of climate change on emerging vector-borne and other infections in the UK', *Environmental Health*, 16(1), pp. 45–51.

Barnes, M. C., Buck, R., Williams, G., Webb, K. and Aylward, M. (2008) 'Beliefs about common health problems and work: A qualitative study', *Social Science and Medicine*, 67, pp. 657–665.

Beaglehole, R. and Bonita, R. (2010) 'What is global health?', *Global Health Action*, 3, pp. 1–2.

Bebber, D.P., Holmes, T. and Gurr, S.J. (2014) 'The global spread of crop pests and pathogens', *Global Ecology and Biogeography*, 23(12), pp. 1398–1407.

Beggs, P. J., Zhang, Y., McGushin, A., Trueck, S., Linnenluecke, M. K., Bambrick, H., Capon, A. G., Vardoulakis, S., Green, D. and Malik, A. (2022) 'The 2022 report of the mja–lancet countdown on health and climate change: Australia unprepared and paying the price', *Medical Journal of Australia*, 217, pp. 439–458.

Behbehani, A. M. (1983) 'The smallpox story: Life and death of an old disease', *Microbiological Reviews*, 47, pp. 455–509.

Birn, A.-E., Pillay, Y. and Holtz, T. H. (2017) *Textbook of Global Health*. Oxford: Oxford University Press.

Bradbury-Jones, C. and Clark, M. (2017) 'Globalisation and global health: Issues for nursing', *Nursing Standard*, 31(39), pp. 54–63.

Browning, M. H., Rigolon, A. and McAnirlin, O. (2022) 'Where greenspace matters most: A systematic review of urbanicity, greenspace, and physical health', *Landscape and Urban Planning*, 217, pp. 1–13.

Buck, R., Barnes, M. C., Cohen, D. and Aylward, M. (2010) 'Common health problems, yellow flags and functioning in a community setting', *Journal of Occupational Rehabilitation*, 20, pp. 235–246.

Castelli, F. (2018) 'Drivers of migration: Why do people move?', *Journal of Travel Medicine*, 25, pp. 1–7.

Chami, R., Hakura, D. and Montiel, P. J. (2009) 'Remittances: An automatic output stabilizer?' Available at: https://papers.ssrn.com/sol3/papers.cfm?abstract_id=1394811 (Accessed: 17 April 2023).

Charlier, P., Claverie, J.M., Sansonetti, P., Coppens, Y., Augias, A., Jacqueline, S., Rengot, F. and Deo, S. (2017) 'Re-emerging infectious diseases from the past: Hysteria or real risk?', *European Journal of Internal* Medicine, 44, pp. 28–30.

Church, D. L. (2004) 'Major factors affecting the emergence and re-emergence of infectious diseases', *Clinics in Laboratory Medicine*, 24, pp. 559–586.

Claborn, D. M. (2018) 'Introductory chapter: What is global health? Current issues in global health'. Available at: www.intechopen.com/chapters/64096 (Accessed: 17 April 2023).

Collignon, P., Beggs, J.J., Walsh, T.R., Gandra, S. and Laxminarayan, R. (2018) 'Anthropological and socioeconomic factors contributing to global antimicrobial resistance: a univariate and multivariable analysis', *The Lancet Planetary Health*, 2(9), pp. e398–e405.

Cugola, F.R., Fernandes, I.R., Russo, F.B., Freitas, B.C., Dias, J.L., Guimarães, K.P., Benazzato, C., Almeida, N., Pignatari, G.C., Romero, S. and Polonio, C.M., 2016. 'The Brazilian Zika virus strain causes birth defects in experimental models', *Nature*, 534(7606), pp. 267–271.

Dao, A., Yaro, A., Diallo, M., Timbiné, S., Huestis, D., Kassogué, Y., Traoré, A., Sanogo, Z., Samaké, D. and Lehmann, T. (2014). 'Signatures of aestivation and migration in Sahelian malaria mosquito populations', *Nature*, 516, pp. 387–390.

Dasgupta, S., Laplante, B., Meisner, C., Wheeler, D. and Yan, J. (2009). 'The impact of sea level rise on developing countries: A comparative analysis', *Climatic Change*, 93, pp. 379–388.

De Cock, K. M., Simone, P. M., Davison, V. and Slutsker, L. (2013). 'The new global health'. Available at: https://stacks.cdc.gov/view/cdc/19160 (Accessed: 17 April 2023).

De Haas, H. (2011). 'The determinants of international migration', Available at: https://ora.ox.ac.uk/objects/uuid:0b10d9e8-810e-4f49-b76f-ba4d6b1faa86 (Accessed: 17 April 2023).

Department of Health. (2011) 'Health is global: An outcomes framework for global health 2011–2015'. Available at: https://assets.publishing.service.gov.uk/government/uploads/system/uploads/attachment_data/file/215656/dh_125671.pdf. (Accessed: 17 April 2023).

Dherani, M., Pope, D., Mascarenhas, M., Smith, K. R., Weber, M. and Bruce, N. (2008) 'Indoor air pollution from unprocessed solid fuel use and pneumonia risk in children aged under five years: A systematic review and meta-analysis', *Bulletin of the World Health Organization*, 86, pp. 390–398.

Đukić, M. and Bodroža, D. (2022) 'Diaspora contribution to the economic development of the republic of Serbia: Remittances and investments'. Available at: http://ebooks.ien.bg.ac.rs/1797/ (Accessed: 17 April 2023).

Dumett, R. E. (1968) 'The campaign against malaria and the expansion of scientific medical and sanitary services in British west Africa, 1898–1910', *African Historical Studies*, 1(2), pp. 153–197.

Edna Ateboh, P. and Raimi, M. O. (2018). 'Corporate civil liability and compensation regime for environmental pollution in the Niger Delta', *International Journal of Recent Advances in Multidisciplinary Research*, 5(06), pp. 3870–3893.

El-Sayed, A. and Kamel, M. (2020) 'Climatic changes and their role in emergence and re-emergence of diseases', *Environmental Science and Pollution Research*, 27, pp. 22336–22352.

Faronbi, J., Ajadi, A. and Gobbens, R. (2020) 'Associations of chronic illnesses and socio-demographic factors with health-related quality of life of older adults in Nigeria: A cross-sectional study', *Ghana Medical Journal*, 54, pp. 164–172.

Faronbi, J., Akinyoola, O., Faronbi, G., Adegbola, G. and Bello, C. (2019) 'Health needs and health seeking behaviour of internally displaced persons in dalori camp, maiduguri, borno state, nigeria', *Research Journal of Health Sciences*, 7, pp. 246–255.

Gelb, S., Kalantaryan, S., McMahon, S. and Perez-Fernandez, M. (2021). *Diaspora Finance for Development: From Remittances to Investment*. Luxembourg: Publications Office of the European Union Luxembourg.

Gu, H., Yan, W., Elahi, E. and Cao, Y. (2020) 'Air pollution risks human mental health: An implication of two-stages least squares estimation of interaction effects'. *Environmental Science and Pollution Research*, 27, pp. 2036–2043.

Hanjra, M.A. and Qureshi, M.E. (2010) 'Global water crisis and future food security in an era of climate change', *Food Policy*, 35(5), pp. 365–377.

Henderson, M., Harvey, S. B., Øverland, S., Mykletun, A. & Hotopf, M. (2011). 'Work and common psychiatric disorders'. Journal of the Royal Society of Medicine, 104, 198–207.

Hirsch, L. A. & Martin, R. (2022). *LSHTM and Colonialism: A Report on the Colonial History of the London School of Hygiene & Tropical Medicine (1899–c. 1960)*. Available at: www.lshtm.ac.uk/research/centres/centre-history-public-health/news/352926/lshtm-and-colonialism-report-colonial-history-london-school-hygiene-tropical [Accessed 7 July 2023].

Hoff, J. (2015). *'Think Globally, Act Locally': Climate Change Mitigation and Citizen Participation. Community Governance and Citizen-Driven Initiatives in Climate Change Mitigation*. Routledge.

Holst, J. (2020). 'Global health – emergence, hegemonic trends and biomedical reductionism'. *Globalization and Health*, 16, 1–11.

Huestis, D. L., Dao, A., Diallo, M., Sanogo, Z. L., Samake, D., Yaro, A. S., Ousman, Y., Linton, Y.-M., Krishna, A. & Veru, L. (2019). 'Windborne long-distance migration of malaria mosquitoes in the sahel', *Nature*, 574, 404–408.

Hujale, M. (2022) 'Somalis abandon their homes in search of food, water and aid as drought deepen. UK: UNHCR, the UN Refugee Agency'. Available at: www.unhcr.org/uk/news/stories/

2022/9/633419134/somalis-abandon-homes-search-food-water-aid-drought-deepens.html (Accessed: 17 April 2023).

Ikonen, N., Savolainen-Kopra, C., Enstone, J. E., Kulmala, I., Pasanen, P., Salmela, A., Salo, S., Nguyen-Van-Tam, J. S. and Ruutu, P. (2018) 'Deposition of respiratory virus pathogens on frequently touched surfaces at airports', *BMC Infectious Diseases*, 18, pp. 1–7.

Ilic, I., Zivanovic Macuzic, I. and Ilic, M. (2022) 'Global outbreak of human monkeypox in 2022: Update of epidemiology', *Tropical Medicine and Infectious Disease*, 7, pp. 264–274.

International Council of Nurses (2022) 'Sustain and retain in 2022 and beyond Geneva'. Available at: www.icn.ch/news/new-report-calls-global-action-plan-address-nursing-workforce-crisis-and-prevent-avoidable (Accessed 16 April 2023).

International Council of Nurses. (2021) 'International council of nurses calls for ethical recruitment process to address critical shortage of nurses'. Available at: www.icn.ch/news/international-council-nurses-calls-ethical-recruitment-process-address-critical-shortage (Accessed: 17 April 2023).

Jonathan, J., Ivoke, N., Aguzie, I. and Nwani, C. (2018) 'Effects of climate change on malaria morbidity and mortality in Taraba state, Nigeria', *African Zoology*, 53, pp. 119–126.

Jones, C. B. and Sherwood, G. (2014) 'The globalization of the nursing workforce: Pulling the pieces together', *Nursing Outlook*, 62, pp. 59–63.

Kahn, L. H., Kaplan, B., Monath, T., Woodall, J. and Conti, L. (2014) 'A manifesto for planetary health', *The Lancet*, 383, p. 1459.

Kan, H., Chen, R. and Tong, S. (2012). 'Ambient air pollution, climate change, and population health in China', *Environment International*, 42, pp. 10–19.

Keesing, F., Belden, L.K., Daszak, P., Dobson, A., Harvell, C.D., Holt, R.D., Hudson, P., Jolles, A., Jones, K.E., Mitchell, C.E. and Myers, S.S. (2010) 'Impacts of biodiversity on the emergence and transmission of infectious diseases', *Nature*, 468(7324), pp. 647–652.

Kingma, M. (2018) *Nurses on the Move: Migration and the Global Health Care Economy*. New York: Cornell University Press.

Koplan, J.P., Bond, T.C., Merson, M.H., Reddy, K.S., Rodriguez, M.H., Sewankambo, N.K. and Wasserheit, J.N. (2009). 'Towards a common definition of global health', *The Lancet*, 373, pp. 1993–1995.

Laville, S. (2020) 'Air pollution a cause in girl's death, coroner rules in landmark case', *The Guardian*. Available at: www.theguardian.com/environment/2020/dec/16/girls-death-contributed-to-by-air-pollution-coroner-rules-in-landmark-case (Accessed: 17 April 2023).

Lenzen, M., Malik, A., Li, M., Fry, J., Weisz, H., Pichler, P.P., Chaves, L.S.M., Capon, A. and Pencheon, D. (2020) 'The environmental footprint of health care: a global assessment', *The Lancet Planetary Health*, 4(7), pp. e271–e279.

Li, H., Nie, W. and Li, J. (2014) 'The benefits and caveats of international nurse migration', *International Journal of Nursing Sciences*, 1, pp. 314–317.

Lim, S.S., Allen, K., Bhutta, Z. A., Dandona, L., Forouzanfar, M. H., Fullman, N., Gething, P. W., Goldberg, E. M., Hay, S. I. and Holmberg, M. (2016). 'Measuring the health-related sustainable development goals in 188 countries: A baseline analysis from the global burden of disease study 2015', *The Lancet*, 388, pp. 1813–1850.

Lipp, E.K., Huq, A. and Colwell, R.R. (2002). 'Effects of global climate on infectious disease: The cholera model', *Clinical Microbiology Reviews*, 15, pp. 757–770.

Lorenzo, F.M.E., Galvez-Tan, J., Icamina, K. and Javier, L. (2007) 'Nurse migration from a source country perspective: Philippine country case study', *Health Services Research*, 42, pp. 1406–1418.

Ma, W., Kahn, R.E. and Richt, J.A. (2009) 'The pig as a mixing vessel for influenza viruses: Human and veterinary implications', *Journal of Molecular and Genetic Medicine*, 3(1), pp. 158–166.

MacLeod, R. and Lewis, M.J. (2022) *Disease, Medicine and Empire: Perspectives on Western Medicine and the Experience of European Expansion*. London: Routledge.

Majra, J. and Gur, A. (2009) 'Climate change and health: Why should India be concerned?', *Indian Journal of Occupational and Environmental Medicine*, 13(1), pp. 11–16.

Manisalidis, I., Stavropoulou, E., Stavropoulos, A. and Bezirtzoglou, E. (2020) 'Environmental and health impacts of air pollution: A review'. *Frontiers in Public Health*, 14, pp. 1–13.

Manyazewal, T. (2017) 'Using the world health organization health system building blocks through survey of healthcare professionals to determine the performance of public healthcare facilities', *Archives of Public Health*, 75, pp. 1–8.

Marchioro, V.S., Benin, G., Meira, D., Meier, C., Olivoto, T., Klein, L.A., Woyann, L.G., Toebe, M. and Bozi, A.H., (2023) 'A scientometric view of wheat blast: the new catastrophic threat to wheat worldwide', *Journal of Plant Pathology*, 105(1), pp. 121–128.

Marques da Costa, E. and Kállay, T. (2020) 'Impacts of green spaces on physical and mental health'. Available at: https://urbact.eu/impacts-green-spaces-physical-and-mental-health-thematic-report (Accessed: 17 April 2023).

McMichael, A. J. and Butler, C. D. (2006) 'Emerging health issues: The widening challenge for population health promotion', *Health Promotion International*, 21, pp. 15–24.

McMichael, A. J., Woodruff, R. E. and Hales, S. (2006) 'Climate change and human health: Present and future risks', *The Lancet*, 367, pp. 859–869.

NHS England. (2022) 'Delivering a "net zero" national health service'. Available: www.england.nhs.uk/greenernhs/wp-content/uploads/sites/51/2022/07/B1728-delivering-a-net-zero-nhs-july-2022.pdf.

Ogunrinde, A. T., Oguntunde, P. G., Akinwumiju, A. S., Fasinmirin, J. T., Olasehinde, D. A., Pham, Q. B., Linh, N. T. T. and Anh, D. T. (2022) 'Impact of climate change and drought attributes in Nigeria'. *Atmosphere*, 13, pp. 1–13.

Olagunju, T., Adewoye, S., Adewoye, A. and Opasola, O. (2021) 'Climate change impacts on environment: Human displacement and social conflicts in Nigeria'. Available at: https://iopscience.iop.org/article/10.1088/1755-1315/655/1/012072/meta (Accessed: 17 April 2023).

Otu, A., Ameh, S., Osifo-Dawodu, E., Alade, E., Ekuri, S. and Idris, J. (2018) 'An account of the Ebola virus disease outbreak in Nigeria: Implications and lessons learnt', BMC *Public Health*, 18, pp. 1–8.

Padhy, S. K., Sarkar, S., Panigrahi, M. and Paul, S. (2015) 'Mental health effects of climate change', *Indian Journal of Occupational and Environmental Medicine*, 1, pp. 3–7.

Pavlović, T.V. and Đorđević, D. (2022) '"Xylella is the enemy that must be fought": Representations of the X. fastidiosa bacterium in the media discourse', *Corpus Pragmatics*, 6(4), pp. 291–306.

Philipsborn, R. P., Sheffield, P., White, A., Osta, A., Anderson, M. S. and Bernstein, A. (2021) 'Climate change and the practice of medicine: Essentials for resident education', *Academic Medicine*, 96, pp. 355–367.

Robertson, R., Gregory, S. and Jabbal, J. (2014) 'The social care and health systems of nine countries'. Available at: https://commed.vcu.edu/IntroPH/Community_Assessment/2014/commission-background-paper-social-care-health-system-other-countries.pdf (Accessed: 17 April 2023).

Saeed, F., Chaudhry, U.K., Raza, A., Charagh, S., Bakhsh, A., Bohra, A., Ali, S., Chitikineni, A., Saeed, Y., Visser, R.G. and Siddique, K.H. (2023) 'Developing future heat-resilient vegetable crops', *Functional & Integrative Genomics*, 23(1), pp. 1–23.

Salvage, J. and White, J. (2020) 'Our Future is Global: Leadership in Nursing and Global Health', *Revista Latino-Americana de Enfermagem*, 28, pp. 1–7.

Shabani, S. (2021) 'A mechanistic view on the neurotoxic effects of air pollution on central nervous system: Risk for autism and neurodegenerative diseases', *Environmental Science and Pollution Research*, 28, pp. 6349–6373.

Sharma, N. (2020). 'The global covid-19 pandemic and the need to change who we think "we" are', *Theory and Event*, 23, 1–11.

Shen, M., Gao, J., Liang, Z., Wang, Y., Du, Y. and Stallones, L. (2015). 'Parental migration patterns and risk of depression and anxiety disorder among rural children aged 10–18 years in China: A cross-sectional study', *BMJ open*, 5, pp. 1–8.

Shepherd, E. (2019). 'Hand in glove: Could your use of disposable gloves cause more harm than good?' Nursing Times. Available at: www.nursingtimes.net/opinion/hand-glove-use-disposable-gloves-cause-harm-good-30-08-2019/ (Accessed: 17 April 2023).

Thapa, D. K., Visentin, D., Kornhaber, R. and Cleary, M. (2018) 'Migration of adult children and mental health of older parents "left behind": An integrative review', *PloS one*, 13, pp. 1–30.

Titler, M. G. (2008) 'The evidence for evidence-based practice implementation. Patient safety and quality: An evidence-based handbook for nurses'. Available at: www.ncbi.nlm.nih.gov/books/NBK2659/ (Accessed: 17 April 2023).

Titus, T., Robertson, D., Sankey, J. B., Mastin, L. and Rengers, F. (2023) 'A review of common natural disasters as analogs for asteroid impact effects and cascading hazards', *Natural Hazards*, 116, pp. 1–48.

Tola, M., Ajibola, O., Idowu, E. T., Omidiji, O., Awolola, S. T. & Amambua-Ngwa, A. (2020). 'Molecular detection of drug resistant polymorphisms in plasmodium falciparum isolates from southwest, Nigeria', *BMC Research Notes*, 13, pp. 1–7.

Ukaogo, P. O., Ewuzie, U. & Onwuka, C. V. (2020) 'Environmental pollution: Causes, effects, and the remedies'. Available at: https://reader.elsevier.com/reader/sd/pii/B9780128190012000218?token=C8F5EB5846FEE5723F9947B7C2EBF58ED568F416A6BC9C2E670BA9D7B2C3ABF1199536609B4C448AB26607E60BBDD0C1&originRegion=eu-west-1&originCreation=20230417145042 (Accessed 17 April 2023).

United Nations. (2016) 'Change begins with me campaign'. Available at: https://sustainabledevelopment.un.org/partnership/?p=13038 (Accessed 1 December 2022).

United Nations (2020) 'The climate crisis – a race we can win'. Available at: www.un.org/sites/un2.un.org/files/2020/01/un75_climate_crisis.pdf [Accessed: 7 July 2023].

United Nations General Assembly (2015) Transforming our world: the 2030 Agenda for Sustainable Development. Available at: https://documents-dds-ny.un.org/doc/UNDOC/GEN/N15/291/89/PDF/N1529189.pdf?OpenElement [Accessed: 7 July 2023].

Valtolina, G. G. and Colombo, C. (2012) 'Psychological well-being, family relations, and developmental issues of children left behind', *Psychological reports*, 111, pp. 905–928.

Waitzman, E. (2022) 'Staff shortages in the NHS and social care sectors'. Available at: https://lordslibrary.parliament.uk/staff-shortages-in-the-nhs-and-social-care-sectors/ (Accessed: 17 April 2023)

Wang, Y.-J., He, B. Y., Fang, L.-H. and Li, H. J. (2011) 'Preliminary study on the health status among the "left-behind" children in the Xiantao rural area of Hubei province', *Chinese Journal of Contemporary Pediatrics*, 13, pp. 977–980.

Waxa, C. (2020) 'Exploring the use of social media to enhance public engagement during times of crisis in the city of Cape Town'. Available at: https://etd.cput.ac.za/handle/20.500.11838/3437 (Accessed: 17 April 2023).

Wilson, M. E. (1995) 'Travel and the emergence of infectious diseases', *Emerging infectious diseases,* 1(2): 39–46.

Worboys, M. (2000) 'The colonial world as mission and mandate: Leprosy and empire, 1900–1940', *Osiris*, 15, pp. 207–218.

World Bank. (2005) 'Global economic prospects 2006: Economic implications of remittances and migration'. Available at: https://elibrary.worldbank.org/doi/abs/10.1596/978-0-8213-6344-7 (Accessed 17 April 2023).

World Health Organization (1978) 'Primary health care: Report of the international conference on primary health care'. Available at: https://apps.who.int/iris/handle/10665/39228 (Accessed: 17 April 2023)

World Health Organization (2008) 'Global malaria control and elimination: Report of a technical review'. Available at: https://apps.who.int/iris/handle/10665/43903 (Accessed 17 April 2023).

World Health Organization (2013a) 'The economics of the social determinants of health and health inequalities: A resource book'. Available at: https://apps.who.int/iris/handle/10665/84213 (Accessed: 17 April 2023)

World Health Organization (2013b) 'Health 2020: A European policy framework supporting action across government and society for health and well-being'. Available at: https://apps.who.int/iris/handle/10665/131300 (Accessed 17 April 2023).

Zhang, H., Wang, W.-X., Lin, C.-J., Feng, X.-B., Shi, J.-B., Jiang, G.-B. and Larssen, T. (2022). 'Decreasing mercury levels in consumer fish over the three decades of increasing mercury emissions in China', *Eco-Environment and Health*, 1, pp. 46–52.

8 Leadership and Management Pillar

Richard Kyle, Anca Ichim, Leila Morgan, Amy Miles, Nikole Petrova, and Barbara Sweeney

Introduction

Effective leadership and management are essential for the advancement of all aspects of nursing practice, education, and research. Student nurses may initially feel unprepared to assume the responsibilities of leaders and managers. They may believe, perhaps, that these roles are for nurses with more experience? Or for those who have a specific job title? Alternatively, as a student nurse, you may relish opportunities to assume leadership roles as you progress through your nurse education programme, influencing others and leading by example? Or perhaps you have not, thus far, given much thought to the meaning of, and difference between, leadership and management?

Students' journey to nurse leadership and management begins from the moment they step onto a nurse education programme. They have experience as managers albeit, initially, of their own learning. Nurse leadership experience begins when students assume responsibilities as representatives of, and ambassadors for, a trusted profession. Student learning is enhanced by input from, and the example of, colleagues in health and social care practice and also in universities and colleges of nurse education. Educators, therefore, play an important role in preparing students to assume leadership and management responsibilities.

This chapter introduces the leadership and management pillar. It is designed to guide professional development as a nurse leader and manager and to explore how effective leadership and management supports excellence in health and social care. We introduce an anonymised scenario from a nurse education context, which demonstrates how students and nurse educators enact leadership and management which enables others to learn and develop professionally.

Following the scenario, we introduce and apply theoretical perspectives regarding this pillar of learning by explaining what constitutes leadership and management and the distinctions between these terms. We summarise some of the, historically, more common approaches to leadership and management styles, namely, autocratic, democratic, and laissez-faire leadership. There is an increasing number of perspectives on leadership in the literature, however, space permits engagement with a limited number which are applicable to nursing practice and education, namely, transactional, transformational, and authentic leadership.

DOI: 10.4324/9781003390565-8

Scenario

Melanie is an experienced registered nurse with over 15 years of clinical experience in acute and emergency nursing. Seven years ago, Melanie joined the university as a simulation lead, focusing on curriculum design, planning, co-ordinating, and evaluating clinical skills and simulation education. Melanie is line-manager to two of the team's less experienced educators, George and Mia, who recently transitioned from clinical to lecturer roles on the undergraduate nurse education programme.

Melanie is aware that both George and Mia bring a wealth of clinical experience to the nurse education programme, but she is concerned that both find the transition to university roles challenging. They have expressed, at times, their desire to return to clinical practice to regain their clinical credibility.

Melanie understands that a successful transition from practice to higher education can be achieved with appropriate support. She reassures George and Mia that the transition from clinical expert to lecturer is gradual. To support Mia and George, Melanie suggests extending their mentorship period to allow them more time to adjust to their new role. She also encourages Mia and George to consider peer mentoring as this is an effective means to support the transition from practice to education. Melanie is committed to ensuring that all members of the clinical skills and simulation team feel valued and are supported as they develop their careers in higher education.

Feedback received from previous teaching sessions demonstrate that students find the simulation sessions valuable to rehearse practice skills. They requested more simulation scenarios will allow them to practice skills in a non-threatening environment.

Therefore, for today's session, Melanie invited final year student nurses to deliver and supervise a Basic Life Support simulation for second-year students in the simulation suite. In partnership with Mia and George, the final year students developed a simulation scenario for the second-year students. Mia and George would deliver the debrief at the end of the simulation. This was the first time they had delivered a simulation debriefing session, however, they had previously observed Melanie deliver a similar session. They are both excited and anxious to be observed by Melanie, their line manager, and to have feedback shared at the end of the session.

The student-facilitated simulation session was designed and planned some months previously as a project for final year providing opportunities to develop their own leadership skills. They had the opportunity to practise and develop strategies to respond to challenges, before delivering their scenarios to the second-year student nurses. The simulation sessions utilise video recording which enables students and lecturers to go back, revisit and reflect, and establish the key learning points to inform future educational practice.

Mia and George know that the significant part of learning from simulation happens in the debriefing stage, where participants can recall and re-evaluate their performance. They reflect on their decision-making and performance during the simulation session. They have chosen the PEARLS (Promoting Excellence and Reflective Learning in Simulation) model to structure their reflection and are aware of research which supports the importance of creating a safe psychological space where participants can engage with learning, reflect and learn.

Distinctions between Management and Leadership

'Leadership' and 'management' are terms that are often used interchangeably and, while there is overlap, there are also important differences between the two terms and practices. Management consultant Peter Drucker's alleged quotation 'Management is doing things right; leadership is doing the right things' (Covey, 1989, p. 101) invites reflection on the distinction. Matt Gavin (2019) from the Harvard Business School, draws on the work of Professors Nancy Koehn, Joe Fuller, and John Kotter to illuminate the differences. He cites John Kotter's definition of leadership:

> the creation of positive, non-incremental change, including the creation of a vision to guide that change – a strategy – the empowerment of people to make the vision happen despite obstacles, and the creation of a coalition of energy and momentum that can move that change forward.
>
> (Gavin, 2019)

Joe Fuller contrasts this with a view of management:

> Management is getting the confused, misguided, unmotivated and misdirected to accomplish a common purpose on a regular, recurring basis . . . The common intersection between leadership and management is an appreciation for what motivates and causes individuals to behave the way they do, and the ability to draw out the best of them with a purpose in mind.
>
> (Gavin, 2019)

Readers are likely to be challenged by Fuller's perspective on management, citing experiences that those managed are generally not 'confused, misguided' or 'unmotivated'. However further elaboration on the distinction between leadership and management, which forms part of the Harvard discussion, may be more illuminating. Gavin (2019) refers to three areas of difference: process versus vision; organising versus aligning; and position versus quality.

(i) *Process versus vision* – Leaders focus on a vision which guides change, on future planning and on creating and embracing opportunities. Managers focus on the achievement of goals through organisational processes relating to, for example, staffing, budgeting and restructuring.

(ii) *Organising versus aligning* – Managers focus on the pursuit of goals through processes, coordinated actions including organising people, to achieve outcomes. Leaders, it is suggested, focus less on organising people and more on exploring ways to influence and align people with a vision, aiming to empower and inspire.

(iii) *Position versus quality* – Whereas 'manager' is a position with a title, role (for example, ward manager) and range of responsibilities, 'leader' has 'a more fluid meaning. It is pointed out that being a manager does not make you a leader – 'The best managers are leaders, but the two are not synonymous. Leadership is the result of action. If you act in a way that inspires, encourages, or engages others, you are a leader. It doesn't matter your title or position' (Gavin, 2019).

Nikole Petrova, student author of this chapter, shared her observations of leaders and managers from her experience of observing nursing practice. She agreed that both managers and leaders had power, both had responsibilities and both 'had to be good at problem-solving', however, she thought there were differences:

> Managers are there to manage resources and make things fair, however, leaders create opportunities for equity . . . Managers are those who tell people what to do, whereas leaders show and teach you how to do it.

Rarely, though, is there a clear distinction between leadership and management in nursing. As our goal is to strive for excellence in health and social care, this means doing the right things right. We need to lead and manage at the same time, carefully finding a balance between a focus on management or leadership for any given situation or group. As we assume more responsibility within our organisations, we need to develop our skills as both managers and leaders, and, crucially, know when to manage more or lead more. We turn next to well established and historical perspectives on leadership.

Foundations of Leadership Theory

There are many different ideas about what makes a good leader. For some, good leaders are individuals who recognise the skills and talents of their team, enabling staff autonomy to independently complete tasks. For others, good leaders inspire their team to maintain focus on an ambitious goal or mission. Some others prefer something in between, with good leadership involving goal setting, checking in regularly to support progress, and making adaptions when necessary. It can help to think about which of these three approaches resonates with you? Which type of leader do you prefer to work with? Which style of leadership do you aspire to adopt? Or which alternative types of leadership are you aware of and are drawn to?

Historically, Western leadership theory was built on the foundation of three leadership styles. As World War II broke out in Europe, psychologists Kurt Lewin, Ronald Lippitt, and Ralph White published their now classic leadership study (Lewin, Lippitt, and White, 1939). Six years earlier, Lewin had fled his home in Germany, increasingly troubled by the rise of fascism as Adolf Hitler acceded to power. Arriving in America, Lewin and his colleagues set about trying to answer a prescient question: 'what underlies such differing patterns of group behaviour as rebellion against authority, persecution of a scapegoat, apathetic submissiveness to authoritarian domination, or attack upon an outgroup?' (Lewin, Lippitt, and White, 1939, p. 271). Incomprehension regarding the persecution and purges happening in his homeland and of the Holocaust to come, are palpable in Lewin's line of enquiry.

To understand how specific leadership styles shape behaviour, Lewin and his colleagues ran an experiment. Ten-year-old boys attended a club where leaders adopted one of three different leadership styles:

- **Authoritarian** – leaders directed the overall task to be completed by the boys step-by-step and decided who each boy would work with.
- **Democratic** – boys and leaders discussed the activities to be done, boys sought guidance from leaders as needed and decided who they would work with.
- **Laissez-faire** – boys were allowed to do what they wished, and leaders did not participate in any way.

During the experiment each group of boys transitioned through these leadership styles over a series of weeks. That way they experienced, what Lewin calls, the 'social climate' of each specific leadership style. Lewin and his team observed the effects and found the results fascinating in terms of both productivity and behaviour. Authoritarian and democratic groups were more productive than the laissez-faire group although when leaders left the room work stopped only in the authoritarian groups. Boys in authoritarian groups fell into one of two patterns of behaviour: apathetic submissiveness or open aggressiveness. This included the persecution of others. Democratic groups, in contrast, were co-operative, enjoyable, and preferred by the boys (Scheidlinger, 1994). Despite the gender and cultural bias in this work towards boys' responses within a specific context, these findings from Lewin and his colleagues' seminal study have profoundly shaped leadership thinking in two ways.

First, the preference for democratic leadership styles. Certainly, there are times in health and social care settings when authoritarian leadership styles are more appropriate. Think, for example, of emergency response situations where clear protocols are activated, leaders are designated to direct activities, allocate people and resources, and redeploy staff from their usual roles if required. Emergency situations such as resuscitation responses to cardiac arrest come to mind.

In other circumstances, nurses acting as autonomous and critical thinking professionals are often left to their own devices to plan and deliver care, with limited direction or supervision, especially in remote and rural community practice. That said, the preference for democratic leadership styles has become a central tenet of current approaches to leadership, and indeed current leadership preferences among Millennials (Faller and Gogek, 2019). We see this in staff surveys that ask nurses how involved they feel in decision-making in their team, or the ubiquity of staff consultation during processes of organisational change (National Health Service, 2023).

Second, Lewin's work highlights the fact that leaders shape the climate of the organisations they work in. Through their actions they change behaviours – for better or worse. We intuitively know this from our own experience. Reflect back on which leadership style you were drawn to. Is your preference shaped by how you feel or act when working with a leader exhibiting this style? Sadly, we see this too in evidence, from reports of care failings (as illustrated in Chapter 3), such as the Francis report into Mid-Staffordshire NHS Foundation Trust. Insights from social psychology draws attention to leadership failings in other contexts, such as in research and the military (Zimbardo, 2014). These show how leadership behaviours set the culture of organisations. Leaders can establish cultures of secrecy and silence, or support people to openly speak up and learn from failure as they strive for excellence in health and social care. It is because leadership styles influence how others behave that understanding how you want to lead is so important. And the good news is individuals have choices regarding the style of leadership they adopt.

Trait-Based Leadership Theories

In the aftermath of World War II, the problem that Lewin and his colleagues foresaw in the research question guiding their boys' club study became a broader concern in leadership thinking: How could leaders like Hitler, Stalin, and Mussolini lead with such conviction that they could motivate people to torture, murder, maim, and disregard the dignity of other humans?

Trait-based leadership theories offered a possible explanation. According to this line of thinking, leaders had innate characteristics – traits – ideally suited to leadership. Qualities such as charisma, decisiveness, determination, intuition, and extroversion. This 'Great Man' theory (so-called because being a man was also invariably one of the inherent traits) shaped thinking for decades. Leaders, so the theory ran, were born, not made.

Trait-based leadership theories sparked attempts to find ever more refined ways of identifying and testing for the exact traits that predisposed people to leadership. Indeed, one of the recommendations in response to the care failings exposed at Mid Staffordshire was that the 'Nursing and Midwifery Council, working with Universities, should consider the introduction of an aptitude test to be undertaken by aspirant registered nurses at entry into the profession, exploring, in particular, candidates' attitudes towards caring, compassion and other necessary professional values' (Francis, 2013, p. 105). Student selection approaches which prioritised compassion and caring would, it was suggested, ensure only those with 'right' traits would start nurse education, as part of a drive towards values-based recruitment. Research has shown, however, that the assumption that values-based recruitment improves recruitment of individuals aligned with organisational values and healthcare quality is unfounded (Spilsbury, 2022).

Trait-based approaches to leadership have been heavily challenged for three main reasons. First, they are *individualistic*. They invest leadership in a single person, rather than a team of people leading together who each bring different values, opinions and professional perspectives to the table. Second, they are *deterministic*. They assume that a fixed set of characteristics naturally result in someone having the aptitude to lead, rather than considering the ways that leadership is a learned behaviour, carefully developed over time. Third, they are *static*. They presume that leadership traits are immutable and that the same set of leadership traits will always be valued in every environment, rather than recognising that leaders may need to adapt their approach to the context in which they lead.

Readers' experience of leading and being led are likely to corroborate this critique. You will have seen that rarely does leadership sit with just one person. You will have witnessed people learning how to lead and growing as leaders around you. And, undoubtedly, you will also have watched how leaders carefully flex their style to respond sensitively to different people and environments.

At the heart of this critique is hope for us all as we step into leadership roles. Although we may not initially think we have the qualities to lead – indeed at times we may feel like imposters – the critique of trait-based theories tells us that we do not lead alone, we can learn how to do it, and we can change our approach.

Transactional and Transformational Theories

The concepts of transactional and transformation leadership help us to think this through more practically (Henry, 2023). *Transactional leadership* focuses on creating structures that support people in organisations to grow. This means implementing organisational policies and processes, including how tasks are delegated, performance is rewarded, and people are treated. Transactional approaches have a greater focus on management – doing things right.

Transformational approaches, on the other hand, are more synonymous with leadership – doing the right things. Transformational approaches focus on vision which encourages the growth of people within the organisation. This involves inspiring staff, embracing ideas and innovation, identifying the needs and passions of your team, and working together to create a shared sense purpose, and proposing a better future that people want to reach with you at the helm. Put another way, transactional approaches tend to focus on sustaining productivity – keeping everything moving forward smoothly. Transformational approaches are about promoting change – embracing innovation, negotiating priorities and enabling engagement.

Motivating people to follow your vision can be challenging. Yet, our exploration of leadership theories gives us some pointers for guidance. Lewin's leadership legacy illustrated that people prefer democratic leadership styles, involving people in making the decisions that shape their future. Critique of the 'great man' myth showed that leaders are made, not born. Learning, adapting, and changing your approach is essential – a critique that is particularly potent in a female-dominated and culturally-diverse profession. This takes us right back to our starting point: the importance of who you uniquely are and how this influences your leadership and management of others. But it also brings us to current leadership thinking in health and social care that has authenticity at its heart and recognises the complex interplay between these values that support cultivation of ethical leadership practices.

Authentic Leadership

Authentic leadership is seen as an emerging leadership style that has the potential to bring positive changes in healthcare settings (Johnson, 2019) by fostering honest relationships (Raso, Fitzpatrick, and Masick, 2020). This builds healthier work environments where staff are supported and encouraged to grow and flourish (Giordano-Mulligan and Eckardt, 2019). According to Gill and Caza (2018), authentic leaders display four core dimensions: self-awareness, transparency, internalised moral perspective and balanced decision-making. Avolio et al. (2004, p. 4) bring even more clarity to the concept and describe authentic leaders as:

> those individuals who are deeply aware of how they think and behave and are perceived by others as being aware of their own and others' values/moral perspective, knowledge, and strengths; aware of the context in which they operate; and who are confident, hopeful, optimistic, resilient, and high on moral character.

The notion of a 'strong leader' can evoke images of strength and confidence, rather than images of vulnerability. However, role modelling vulnerability suggests an openness within a team, which can bring about an overall more honest and collaborative team dynamic (Couris, 2020). Couris (2020) expands upon this further, detailing elements of vulnerability within leadership that will encourage this attitude to flourish within a team: being transparent, asking for feedback, expressing emotions, kindness, shared learning and encouraging others' vulnerability too.

Sharing your vulnerabilities with others, and instilling vulnerability and authenticity within leadership practice, can also often take courage and needs to be approached wisely. Courage, defined as the ability to do something which evokes fear and showing strength in response (Andrews, 2020), needs to be demonstrated with discernment. It can feel risky to allow emotions into your leadership, however, this courage may ultimately influence positive changes in others, as well as wider processes within a team (Brown, 2012). Leaders need, however, to ensure they continue to inspire the trust and confidence of a team and to enable team members, to feel that their leader is morally resilient with their focus directed towards team flourishing and the overall mission to work towards excellence in their chosen field. Student author of this chapter, Nikole Petrova, shared her list of the features of a 'good leader':

A good leader has a long-term plan and brings about change for the greater good and for sustainable healthcare. Someone who is a good problem-solver, who is motivational and who cares about people. A good leader is ready for change, is not afraid to take risks and who thinks outside the box to find solutions. A good leader is someone who is humble, who actions ideas, who is a people's person and a good listener and who leads by example, using latest evidence and who is not afraid to take on a challenge.

Nikole's summary features of a good leader are drawn, primarily, from her experience in healthcare practice, however, they also seem applicable to good leadership in the educational context. We turn to this next.

Educational Leadership

Nurse educators such as Simulation Lead (Melanie) and new lecturers (George and Mia) – as in the scenario above – navigate much complexity as they manage practical educational arrangements and inspire students and colleagues through professional leadership. The styles of leadership outlined above are relevant to the nurse education context, particularly democratic, transformational, transactional and, with discernment, authentic leadership. Nurse educators have responsibilities to ensure the requirements of nurse regulation are met, ensuring that students have opportunities to engage in critical thinking and to develop the knowledge, skills, and values necessary to be fit for nurse registration and for contemporary health and social care practice. Nurse educators also have responsibilities to support and develop team members and to continue their own professional development.

Leadership has been at the centre of influential nursing studies and scholarship since the last century. However, aspects of educational leadership have been less explored (Sandhu, 2019). Leadership in nurse education reflects the interplay of nurse professional and nurse academic identities with ongoing debate regarding priorities between theory and practice and between clinical settings and educational organisations (Van Diggele et al., 2020). The discourse on educational leadership might, therefore, unveil an inner tension between the professional and the academic roles of nurses.

Nurses provide leadership in educating patients and families (Choi, Kim, and Kim, 2018). They naturally lead patients' learning and oversee the health or educational institutions' pedagogical, psychological, and sociological dimensions (Karaman et al., 2023). However, attention needs to be paid to formal educational leadership roles. Ramani et al. (2021), for example, suggested that transitioning from a clinical role to an educational leadership role implies an identity shift. All nurse educators and academics, involved in providing high-quality and meaningful learning experience for nursing students, should reflect on how their leadership skills influence such a crucial formative process.

Both educators and learners need to integrate clinical and educational aspects of their identities by incorporating relevant pedagogic knowledge, skills, and values. They will benefit from engagement with those more experienced to be able to negotiate and sustain the paradigm shift when it occurs. This might imply re-organising their patterns of knowing as they respond to challenges (Van Diggele et al., 2020). However, reflection plays a vital role in educational leadership and educational leaders will benefit from embracing reflective practice, curiosity, humility, and authenticity (Ramani et al., 2021). Fields, Kenny, and Mueller (2019) also argue that educational leadership involves affective skills and dispositions, including humility, during academic work and ordinary life. This can be achieved by establishing trust, building healthy and productive relationships with students, and encouraging honest, open dialogue, regarding teaching and learning (Van Diggele et al., 2020). Another essential aspect of educational leadership is coaching, mentoring, and empowering colleagues, facilitating their learning. This aspect leads to building collegial relationships and understanding local contexts (Fields et al., 2019)

Bolander and Tomson (2017) highlighted other aspects of optimising the educational leader role. These activities (abridged) consisted of having:

> a student-centred perspective, mapping the students and faculty development needs, addressing these needs in an inspirational and effective way, facilitating a creative organizational learning and creating networks, both within the university and with stakeholders.
>
> (Bolander and Tomson, 2017, p. 510)

Finally, a critical aspect of effective educational leadership is creating relationships between educational leaders, including teaching staff, and students. Implementing communities of practice of educational leaders and networking can be pivotal to sustaining the challenges of the nurse education system (Kothari et al., 2015). In addition, improving education and effecting changes in health services can be achieved by providing opportunities for educational leadership development.

Putting Leadership into Practice – Application to Scenario

Through daily actions, reflections and discussions with fellow students, clinical and education teams, students are influencing others and potentially inspiring change. From first encounters with health and social care, student nurses have opportunities to observe, and evaluate, the practice of people in leadership and managerial roles. Judgements will be made regarding good and less good managers, between good and less good leaders. Similarly, experienced and less experienced nurse educators influence others, learn from others and make judgements about management and leadership.

The student-facilitated Basic Life Support (BLS) simulation session in the scenario, involved final year students facilitating the learning of second year students, with support from Mia and George (new nurse lecturers). Registered nurse and Simulation Lead, Melanie, assumed overall leadership and responsibility for the safe and competent organisation and running of the session. She, therefore, had attended to the preparation of George and Mia who were leading the session and of the final year students who were facilitating learning. Melanie had also provided information and reassurance to the second year students, who were receiving the BLS education session. She ensured that Mia and George appreciated the importance of debriefing in simulation activities so participants can recall and re-evaluate their performance. Both lecturers and students benefit from reflecting on their decision-making and performance during the simulation session.

Simulation-based learning is now an established strategy for learning and supporting nursing students in developing technical and non-technical skills and promoting critical thinking, communication, decision making and leadership skills in a non-threatening environment (Kourkouta et al., 2021). Much of the literature praises the role of clinical simulation in fostering leadership skills (Cohen et al., 2019) suggests that team-based simulation can enhance nurses' authentic leadership traits. The student-facilitated simulation has enjoyed much attention in the last few years, with Curtis et al. (2016) reporting high satisfaction and self-confidence among nursing students when the peer-to-peer simulation was used.

The student-facilitated simulation has received much attention in recent years, with Curtis et al. (2016) reporting high satisfaction and self-confidence among nursing students when the peer-to-peer simulation was used. Brown and Rode (2018) suggest that leadership skills are fostered and enhanced by the peer-to-peer facilitation.

As indicated in the scenario, Mia and George selected the PEARLS (Promoting Excellence and Reflective Learning in Simulation) model to structure their reflection. This is a healthcare simulation debriefing tool (Eppich and Cheng, 2015) which enables educators to facilitate aspects of the simulation experience, for example, development of technical skills, clinical decision-making, teamwork, and inter-professional collaboration. Melanie demonstrated democratic leadership as she supported final year students to plan the BLS session, guiding and enabling them to identify key learning outcomes from the curriculum and evidence underpinning best practice in BLS training. Melanie also enabled Mia and George to learn about the importance of simulation debriefing, directing them to learning resources and inviting the, to plan an evidence-based approach to the creation of a safe psychological space where participants can engage safely with learning about the important knowledge skills and values relating to BLS.

Earlier in the chapter, we introduced transactional and transformational leadership. In the context of educational management and leadership, we need to remember *why* leadership and management are important and the direct impact this has on student learning and staff development. National Health Service (2022) discusses the importance of shared decision-making, increasing patient choices and enabling self-care. In nurse education, sensitivity to patient and family involvement must be prioritised. This is a theme that has been discussed at length with the Academy of Nursing's patient and public involvement (PPI) group. Barbara Sweeney, co-author of this chapter and co-chair of our PPI group, said:

> However transactional the care, we must always show compassion and kindness. Talking to an unconscious patient, explaining what you are doing and why, is the right thing and a powerful message, and as leaders we must exhibit these behaviours from the front.

In all simulation education contexts, student nurses need to be reminded of the contextual features of care organisations that can enhance or undermine care practices. For example, the Royal College of Nursing (2023) discusses the right number of nurses with the right skills in the right place and the right time and the impact this can have on patient safety. This involves managerial and leadership considerations that enough nurses are available to provide therapeutic care, and in terms of leadership, can involve highlighting safety concerns when there is an under resourcing of clinical staff.

The discussion of leadership in this chapter needs, therefore, to be enhanced by engagement with the content and reflection stimulated by other pillars. For example, leadership and management in nurse education and practice needs to prioritise fundamentals of care (Chapter 2). Leadership and management in nurse education and practice need to be both evidence-based (see Chapter 4) and values-based, underpinned by ethics and professionalism (Chapter 3). The comment cited above from PPI group member, Barbara Sweeney, reminds of the importance of inviting and listening carefully to insights from patients and families and including their lived experience in nurse education and research (Chapter 5). There needs also to be commitment to respond competently to the physical and mental health and well-being of patients and families on the receiving end of care and support (Chapter 6). Sensitivity is also required in responding to the well-being of students and staff, particularly those new to nurse education, who may require additional guidance and support. The global health pillar of this book (Chapter 7) reminds also that we need to be open-minded and humble regarding learning from other cultural contexts. Research, for example, relating to immersive simulation has inspired some UK nurse educators to include more innovative approaches to the development of ethical care (Gallagher et al., 2017, 2020).

Good leadership and management in nurse education and practice are imperative if we are to succeed in inspiring student nurses and colleagues to aspire to excellence in health and social care. That does not mean, however, that the outcomes will always be favourable. What is important, as suggested by the scenario, is the role of different forms of leadership. There is benefit from: providing senior students, leading less experienced students in the development of new knowledge and skills; new lecturers supporting each other and providing leadership to students; and expert educators, such as Melanie, demonstrating leadership which supports, guides and assumes overall responsibility for educational activity that enables the rehearsal of core skills in a safe, controlled and respectful environment.

Conclusion

Leadership and management are not optional extras in nursing practice and education but are, rather, integral to the practices of nursing, nurse education and research. Effective and ethical leadership and management are essential components of the aspiration to excellence in care. This chapter introduced the background to some well-established approaches to leadership, namely, autocratic, democratic, and laissez-faire approaches. More recent approaches, now included on the leadership repertoire, include transactional, transformational and authentic leadership. These approaches provide insights which illuminate important aspects of leadership and management in nurse education, which has been the focus on this chapter.

The simulation scenario demonstrated the diversity of relationships which are negotiated in innovative nurse education programmes. Students engaged with, and supported the development of, other students. Expert and less experienced educators worked together to provide the best possible education experience for students. The discussion demonstrated the importance of remaining attentive to, and providing support for, nurses who transition from clinical practice to education contexts. The involvement of PPI members reminds of the importance of focusing on the lived experience of patients and families, perspectives which need to be central to nurse education. Implied throughout this chapter, is the importance of leadership and management approaches which serve to inspire curiosity, encourage humility and non-complacency, and prioritise respect and inclusion in nurse education, practice and research.

We give the last word to our final year student chapter author, Nikole Petrova, who shared what she aspires to as a future nurse leader:

I would like to be a humble leader who doesn't boast about her achievements. A leader who leads safe practice, underpinned by evidence, and who motivates others to do the same. I would like to be a leader who is kind to others and who is not afraid to try new ideas. A leader who is OK with failure, as through failure comes learning and innovation.

Takeaways for Student Nurses

- Effective and ethical leadership in nurse education and practice are integral to the aspiration to excellence in health and social care.
- Leadership and management overlap, however, they are not the same. It is important to reflect on each and to consider how they are enacted in nurse education and practice.
- A wide range of approaches to leadership exist, and some are introduced in this chapter. Consider which approach or style you observe in your nursing practice and which you think is most effective and ethical.
- Students have an important part to play in advancing the profession of nursing by acting as ambassadors and role models. Reflect on strategies you might utilise to educate others of the complexity and importance of nursing.
- A commitment to exemplary nurse leadership and management in nurse education, practice and research requires demonstration of curiosity, humility, open-mindedness and respect. This requires ongoing reflection, education and professional development.

Takeaways for educators/practitioners

- Educating and supporting students to be the best they can be as nurse leaders requires reflection and creativity.
- Nurses in practice and in educational contexts serve as role models for students and other members of the multi-professional team.
- Engagement with students and less experienced colleagues requires sensitivity and space to create opportunities for them to contribute positively to practice.
- Incorporating the voices of patients and families in the leadership and management learning opportunities provided to students will greatly enhance their learning.
- The seven pillars of learning pillars introduced in this text are complementary to the knowledge, skills and values you promote in your activities which support student learning and development.
- Remember that your expertise and experience are highly valued and much needed in developing future generations of effective and ethical nurse leaders.

References

Andrews, J. (2020) 'Perspectives: Courage in nursing leadership and innovation', *Journal of Research in Nursing*, 25(3), pp. 308–311.

Avolio, B., Luthans, F. and Walumbwa, F.O. (2004). *Authentic Leadership: Theory-Building for Veritable Sustained Performance*. Working paper. Lincoln: Gallup Leadership Institute, University of Nebraska.

Bolander Laksov, K. and Tomson, T. (2017) 'Becoming an educational leader–exploring leadership in medical education', *International Journal of Leadership in Education*, 20(4), pp. 506–516.

Brown, B. (2012) *Daring Greatly: How the Courage to Be Vulnerable Transforms the Way We Live, Love, Parent, and Lead*. New York: Baker and Taylor.

Brown, K. M. and Rode, J. L. (2018) 'Leadership development through peer-facilitated simulation in nursing education', *Journal of Nursing Education*, 57(1), pp. 53–57.

Choi, E.H., Kim, E.K. and Kim, P.B. (2018) 'Effects of the educational leadership of nursing unit managers on team effectiveness: mediating effects of organizational communication', *Asian Nursing Research*, 12(2), pp. 99–105.

Cohen, D., Vlaev, I., McMahon, L., Harvey, S., Mitchell, A., Borovoi, L. and Darzi, A., (2019) 'The Crucible simulation: behavioral simulation improves clinical leadership skills and understanding of complex health policy change', *Health Care Management Review*, 44(3), pp. 246–255.

Couris, J. D. (2020) 'Vulnerability: The secret to authentic leadership through the pandemic', *Journal of Healthcare Management*, 65(4), pp. 248–251.

Covey, S.R. (1989) *The Seven Habits of Highly Effective People*. London: Simon and Schuster.

Curtis, E., Ryan, C., Roy, S., Simes, T., Lapkin, S., O'Neill, B. and Faithfull-Byrne, A. (2016) 'Incorporating peer-to-peer facilitation with a mid-level fidelity student led simulation experience for undergraduate nurses', *Nurse Education in Practice*, 20, pp. 80–84.

Covey, S.R. (1989) *The Seven Habits of Highly Effective People*. London: Simon and Schuster.

Eppich, W. and Cheng, A. (2015) 'Promoting Excellence and Reflective Learning in Simulation (PEARLS) development and rationale for a blended approach to health care simulation briefing', *Simulation in Healthcare*, 10(2), pp. 106–115.

Faller, M.S. and Gogek J. (2019) 'Break from the past: Survey suggests modern leadership styles needed for millennial nurses' *Nurse Leader*, 17(2), pp. 135–140.

Francis, R. (2013) 'Report of the Mid Staffordshire NHS Foundation Trust public inquiry: Executive summary'. Available at: https://assets.publishing.service.gov.uk/government/uploads/system/uploads/attachment_data/file/279124/0947.pdf 9 Accessed 27 April 2023).

Fields, J., Kenny, N.A. and Mueller, R.A. (2019) 'Conceptualizing educational leadership in an academic development program', *International Journal for Academic Development*, 24(3), pp. 218–231.

Gallagher A., Williams E., Peacock M., Zasada M. and Cox, A. (2020) 'Findings from a mixed methods pragmatic cluster trial evaluating the impact of ethics education interventions on residential care-givers', *Nursing Inquiry*, 28(2), pp. 1–12.

Gallagher A., Peacock M., Zasada M., Coucke T. Cox, A. and Janssens, N. (2017) 'Care-givers' reflections on an ethics education immersive simulation care experience: A series of epiphanous events', *Nursing Inquiry*, 24(3), pp. 1–10.

Gavin, M. (2019) 'Leadership vs. management: What's the difference?' Available at: https://online.hbs.edu/blog/post/leadership-vs-management (Accessed: 27 April 2023).

Gill, C. and Caza, A. (2018) 'An investigation of Authentic Leadership's individual and group influences on follower responses', *Journal of Management*, 44(2), pp. 530–554.

Giordano-Mulligan, M. and Eckardt, S. (2019) 'Authentic nurse leadership conceptual framework', *Nursing Administration Quarterly*, 43(2), pp. 164–174.

Henry, H. (2023) *Be a Leader in Nursing: A Practical Guide for Nursing Students*. London: Elsevier.

Johnson, S. L. (2019) 'Authentic leadership theory and practical applications in nuclear medicine', *Journal of Nuclear Medicine Technology*, 47(3), pp. 181–188.

Karaman, F., KavgaoǦlu, D., Yildirim, G., Rashidi, M., Ünsal Jafarov, G., Zahoor, H. and Kiskaç, N. (2023) 'Development of the educational leadership scale for nursing students: a methodological study', *BMC Nursing*, 22(1), pp. 1–10.

Kothari, A., Boyko, J.A., Conklin, J., Stolee, P. and Sibbald, S.L. (2015) 'Communities of practice for supporting health systems change: a missed opportunity', *Health Research Policy and Systems*, 13(1), pp. 1–9.

Kourkouta, L., Kaptanoglu, A.Y., Koukourikos, K., Iliadis, C. and Ouzounakis, P. (2021) Leadership and teamwork in nursing', *Journal of Healthcare Communications*, 6(22), pp. 1–4.

Lewin, K., Lippitt, R., and White, R.K. (1939) 'Patterns of aggressive behavior in experimentally created "social climates"', *Journal of Social Psychology*, 10(2), pp. 271–299.

National Health Service. (2022) 'Shared decision-making: Summary guide'. Available at: www.england.nhs.uk/publication/shared-decision-making-summary-guide/ (Accessed: 27 April 2023)

National Health Service. (2023) 'NHS staff survey'. Available at: www.nhsstaffsurveys.com/ (Accessed: 27 April 2023).

Ramani, S., McKimm, J., Findyartini, A., Nadarajah, V.D., Hays, R., Chisolm, M.S., Filipe, H.P., Fornari, A., Kachur, E.K., Kusurkar, R.A. and Thampy, H. (2021) 'Twelve tips for developing a global community of scholars in health professions education', *Medical Teacher*, 43(8), pp. 966–971.

Raso, R., Fitzpatrick, J.J. and Masick, K. (2020) 'Clinical nurses' perceptions of authentic nurse leadership and healthy work environment', *JONA: The Journal of Nursing Administration*, 50(9), pp. 489–494.

Royal College of Nursing. (2023) 'Impact of staffing levels on safe and effective patient care: Literature review'. Available at: www.rcn.org.uk/-/media/Royal-College-Of-Nursing/Documents/Publications/2023/February/010-665.pdf (Accessed: 27 April 2023).

Sandhu, D. (2019) 'Healthcare educational leadership in the twenty-first century. Medical Teacher', 41(6), pp. 614–618.

Scheidlinger, S. (1994) 'The Lewin, Lippitt and White study of leadership and "social climates" revisited', *International Journal of Group Psychotherapy*, 44(1), pp. 123–127.

Spilsbury K. (2022) 'Values based recruitment: What works, for whom, why, and in what circumstances?' Available at: https://eprints.whiterose.ac.uk/190125/1/PR-R10-0514-14002_VBR%20FINAL%20REPORT_20%20May%202022.pdf (Accessed: 27 April 2023).

Van Diggele, C., Burgess, A., Roberts, C. and Mellis, C. (2020) 'Leadership in healthcare education', *BMC Medical Education*, 20, pp. 1–6.

Zimbardo, P. (2014) *The Lucifer Effect: How Good People Turn Evil*. London: Ebury Publishing.

9   Integrating the Seven Pillars of Learning: Student Perspectives

Hayley Rich, Charli Morris, Roxanne Kennedy, Nikole Petrova, Bethany Gooding, Matthew Jones, and Isobel Coxon

Introduction

The purpose of this book has been to demonstrate the value and applications of the seven pillars of learning in nursing practice and education. In this chapter, we bring together all of the pillars of nursing and apply them all to a single scenario. The anonymised scenario provides an example of the challenges presented to student nurses and how, by approaching care provision using the pillars, they can navigate these challenges and work towards excellence in care. Whereas previous chapters illustrate how individual pillars relate to a given scenario, this chapter demonstrates how they can be brought together by student nurses to develop and grow their skills, knowledge and values to support them in their careers. It will exemplify how, at every stage of a student nurses' progression, the pillars provide a framework from which to build and advance their practice.

Scenario

Rachel and Ashley are students on an undergraduate pre-registration nurse education programme. They are currently on placement in an oncology ward. Rachel is 45 years old and is in her first year of the programme. Prior to starting the course, she served in the Navy working around the world supporting local communities. She is currently on placement with Ashley, who is 22 years old. Ashley identifies as non-binary, using the pronouns 'they/them', and is in their final year of the nurse education programme. Ashley joined the course immediately after finishing college, as it is a career they have always wanted to pursue.

While working on the ward, a registered nurse allocated responsibility to both students for the provision of care to a patient, Fatima, using the Collaborative Learning in Practice model (CLIP) of practice learning. This model of learning enables peer-to-peer support on placement by students at different stages of their programme. Students organise and deliver care, overseen by a practice supervisor/assessor.

Fatima is a 55-year-old Muslim woman. She lives with her female partner, Yumi. Fatima's parents are unaware of her relationship with Yumi, due to Fatima's concerns about their reaction given their devout faith. Fatima was being treated for breast cancer, with metastases

DOI: 10.4324/9781003390565-9

to her brain, and is now declining further treatment. Treatment options include double mastectomy and craniotomy as well as chemotherapy and radiotherapy.

Rachel was present during a ward round when Fatima and her doctor discussed her care plan. Fatima made it clear she did not want surgery or further treatment. Following this discussion, she signed a treatment escalation plan (TEP) form to allow a natural death with no further active treatment. Fatima was placed on the palliative care pathway and is now seeking hospice care. Rachel is finding Fatima's decision to decline further treatment challenging and has found caring for her difficult. During a CLIP debrief session, Rachel raised these difficulties with Ashley. Rachel acknowledges that Ashley has more experience with palliative care and can support her in her development as a nurse in this aspect of her practice.

Rachel shared with Ashley that she does not understand how a person can 'give up on life when there are so many treatments available'. She says she feels the doctor did not encourage Fatima to seek alternative treatments and just went along with whatever Fatima wanted. Ashley supported Rachel to express her concerns and encouraged her to reflect on why she felt that way. Ashley also encouraged Rachel to reflect on her professional ethics, values and responsibilities, providing examples of situations in which they have found this challenging to their own values and beliefs.

Rachel has, likewise, been able to support Ashley through difficult moments using her life experiences. Ashley has had difficulties, at times, as patients sometimes struggle to understand and wrongly assume their gender. One morning, during the placement, Fatima disclosed to Rachel that she considers Ashley male. She explains that, due to her faith, she can only receive personal care from a female. Rachel explained that Ashley is non-binary, meaning they had no identified gender such as male or female. Although Fatima does not identify as a practicing Muslim, she was raised by devout Muslim parents. As a result, she finds it challenging to receive personal care from Ashley as she still views them as male. Ashley asked Rachel how best to go about supporting Fatima. Rachel has a broader life experience, because of her navy career, and worked closely with Muslim communities abroad. Ashley feels Rachel is well placed to provide support in caring for Fatima. Rachel has been supporting Ashley with this, including providing guidance with negotiating the care provided for Fatima. Rachel and Ashley discuss possible steps such as contacting their equality and diversity team, and the chaplaincy team within the hospital, to provide both they and Fatima with support and guidance with the issues raised.

Fatima is preparing to be transferred to the hospice team and so Rachel and Ashley will shortly no longer be providing care for her, however, the challenges they have identified and addressed in providing care for her will impact on their future practice.

We turn next to the application of the seven pillars learning to this scenario. We explore how insights from the fundamentals of nursing care pillar illuminate the experiences of Rachel and Ashley as they organise and deliver care to Fatima.

Fundamentals of Nursing Care Pillar

Holistic patient care is an established and understood approach in health and social care. According to Selman et al. (2014), this approach directs professionals to provide interventions and care that looks beyond the patient's disease and values the 'whole' person and the patient's environment. Therefore, it is critical that nurses provide holistic care that encompasses the patient's biopsychosocial needs, including both clinical and therapeutic care which includes palliative and end-of-life treatment. In the scenario, Fatima chooses to withdraw from any further cancer treatment and has requested transfer to a hospice for palliative care. After this decision, Fatima was placed on a palliative care pathway, a TEP form was discussed and signed and active treatment was stopped. The therapeutic and communicative care provided by the two nursing students, Ashley and Rachel, to support Fatima with decisions placed Fatima at the centre of her care.

Fatima was able to take control of her care and the outcome of her treatment, which empowered her as she experienced her terminal illness. This reflects the concept of holistic patient care which goes beyond the healing of an illness and recognises the centrality of patient views in the provision of meaningful and good end-of-life care (Selman et al., 2014). In the scenario, Rachel found it difficult to accept Fatima's decision, however, it was essential that Fatima's perspective and point of view was at the forefront of the support provided for her to stop further active treatment. Hence, the role and importance of therapeutic care alongside clinical care in patient health. For Fatima, the decisions made represented comfort and palliative care in a hospice environment rather than active treatment. So, holistic patient care represents health as a state of complete physical, mental and social wellbeing (World Health Organization, 2020), which is different for every patient. To provide holistic care, the patient's voice must be at the centre of their care and treatment. This was evident in the scenario, where Ashley and Rachel discussed Fatima's decision, with her wishes at the forefront of their discussions and the support that was provided to her.

Holistic, person-centred care reflects the therapeutic and task-orientated care that healthcare professionals provide in their practise. Hunter-Jones et al. (2022) discusses how the aim of person-centred care should be provided, based on what is important to the person, from their own perspective. This allows the professional to value the patient's voice and to provide a level of understanding regarding their experiences and care. Fatima's wishes were to receive palliative care in a hospice with no further treatment. Rachel could not understand why the doctor did not encourage Fatima more to pursue active treatment. However, holistic care is a balance between therapeutic and task-orientated care. Holistic care includes dignity, compassion and respect which is facilitated via co-ordinated, enabling personal care (Hunter-Jones et al., 2022). Therefore, it was essential in this scenario that a therapeutic relationship was established with Fatima and promoted through communicative and compassionate support. The physical, social and psychological dimensions involved in the fundamentals of nursing care is mediated via the therapeutic relationships developed between professional and patient (Kitson, Athlin, and Conroy, 2014).

Alongside the development of a therapeutic relationship between Fatima and the student nurses were care assessment, facilitation, and coordination to ensure that Fatima's wishes were respected. Holistic care is an established balance between therapeutic and task-orientated care which is suited to the patient and facilitated by their voice. The fundamentals of care nursing framework (Kitson et al., 2014) demonstrates the importance of the integration of care with the therapeutic relationship at the centre of this framework. This framework depicts the balance among physical, psychosocial and relational dimensions involved in the care of a patient. If the patient's care became unbalanced, care and treatment decisions could have denied Fatima's wishes, placing the professional at the centre of care rather than the patient her/himself.

Spirituality and religion are fundamental aspects of holistic care. Linking back to the scenario, Fatima is not a practising Muslim but was raised by her parents, who are devout Muslims. Fatima expresses her wishes to not receive personal care from Ashley, a student nurse who is non-binary. Batstone and Bailey (2019) highlight the increase of spiritual distress that patient's experience when in hospital. Spiritual suffering is more prevalent during palliative and end-of-life stages. It is critical for every health and social care professional to provide consistent and equal care for every patient as a part of a diverse and multi-cultural society. Spiritual care may differ by context, culture, and patient situation (Batstone and Bailey, 2019). This includes the respect for patient's requests and wishes regarding personal care. Therefore, it is essential that Ashley values and respects Fatima's wishes regarding her personal care. The Nursing and Midwifery Council (2018) code addresses the importance of acceptance, respect, and equality from the patient to the professional. Rachel and Ashley reflect upon this together, in collaboration with Fatima, to coordinate her care which respects patient and students. So, teamwork between patient and professional is essential to provide holistic care that is based upon patient and professional perspectives.

We turn next to reflection on the some of the challenging ethical issues which arise in this scenario and the role of professionalism.

Ethics and Professionalism Pillar

Throughout this scenario, there are significant ethical and professional considerations which impact on the practice of student nurses, Rachel and Ashley. During a student nurses' education journey, many complex clinical encounters with patients are inevitably experienced. These experiences will inescapably influence the quality of care delivered and impact future professional development (Wolf and Langer, 2000; Pedersen and Sivonen, 2012). Supporting the ethical and professional development of student nurses is essential to equip them with the necessary skills to successfully navigate these experiences, avoid burnout, and increase retention (Roach, 2002).

The ethical dilemma, faced by Rachel in the scenario, involves the ethical principles 'respect for autonomy' and 'non-maleficence'. These are two of Beauchamp and Childress's (2019) four principles' approach to biomedical ethics, as discussed in Chapter 3. Rachel's difficulty to accept Fatima's decision to decline curative treatment puts her in a morally challenging position. By respecting Fatima's autonomy and understanding a patient's right to decline, Rachel is attempting to advocate for Fatima and this may reduce her moral distress (Gallagher, 2020).

Ashley's experience with non-binary gender identity, in the scenario, highlights the importance of cultural humility and ethical sensitivity in health and social care. As a nurse, it is important to understand and respect patients' cultural beliefs and preferences, even if they differ from one's own. To successfully navigate ethical dilemmas, such as a patient declining care, nurses must possess the ability to first identify moral challenges, and then reflect upon them both as an individual and as a team. This is a crucial component for the moral development of the student nurse (Musto *et al.*, 2015).

The scenario also stresses the importance of professionalism and the use of codes in nursing practice. Nursing and ethical codes, such as the International Council of Nurses (2021) code and the Nursing and Midwifery Council (2018) code – and similar codes for nurses in other countries – provide guidance and principles for ethical and professional conduct in nursing. Rachel and Ashley's use of reflection and discussion to explore ethical and professional issues, as well as their adherence to their professional Code, highlights their dedication to upholding the principles of nursing professionalism as well as collaboratively engaging in their moral and ethical development. The situation with Fatima's relationship with Yumi raises important considerations around patient confidentiality and privacy. It is required for healthcare professionals to respect patients' privacy and not disclose sensitive information to others, for example parents, without their explicit consent. Maintaining confidentiality prevents jeopardising the well-being of the patient and strengthens trust in the nurse-patient relationship (Fowler, 2021).

Finally, the scenario also highlights the importance of recognising the staff hierarchy present in care settings, and how this can impact professionalism. Pedersen and Sivonen (2012) suggest hierarchy in healthcare can compromise a student nurses' moral integrity if they experience low status, poor recognition, or are prevented from practicing in line with their ethical convictions. In this case, there are aspects of the scenario where both students support each other's learning and moral development, despite Ashley being in her final year, and Rachel in her first year. This demonstrates how students at various levels of education can work together and support each other's learning and development. However, it is important to recognise there is a power dynamic present in healthcare settings, with more experienced professionals having more authority and influence. As such it is essential for all healthcare professionals, regardless of their level of education, to maintain professionalism and respect the boundaries of their roles and responsibilities.

Insights from the ethics and professionalism pillar illuminate important features of the scenario. This focuses on the values underpinning nursing practice and education, what has been described as values-based practice. We turn next to an equally important pillar which relates to evidence-based practice.

Evidence for Practice Pillar

The evidence for practice pillar of learning focuses on evidence-based practice (EBP) which is important when discussing Rachel and Ashley's situation. As discussed in Chapter 4, EBP underpins all aspects of nursing, from the evidence underpinning care assessment, planning, delivery and leadership to the evidence underpinning learning and teaching in nurse education. As with all pillars, the evidence for practice pillar focuses on ensuring that the interests and flourishing of patients, families and communities are prioritised throughout.

Patient-centredness is especially pertinent in Fatima's case. The research and medical investigations that form the evidence for her diagnosis and prognosis, while important, are only one part of the story of her care journey. Upon receiving this information, the next steps for Fatima, focus on respecting her autonomy in relation to her care and the ability of her healthcare team to effectively respect her choices and the decision-making process. It is important to support Fatima and her loved ones in navigating palliative care in a way that is as supportive and respectful as possible. To be able to do this effectively, student nurses like Rachel and Ashley must be taught the importance of patient autonomy during their education and to have a good level of understanding of the International Council of Nurses Code of Ethics (2021). It is important for Rachel and Ashley to draw on evidence of shared decision-making such as in National Institute for Health and Care Excellence (National Institute for Health and Care Excellence, 2020a) when supporting Fatima to ensure she has a good understanding of her prognosis and treatment options, and is able to understand and discuss the potential harms and benefits of different options.

Evidence and nursing practice are fundamentally linked, from formal scientific research to more personal experiences such as navigating the moral challenges of supporting patients during the palliative care pathway. An essential component of research into effective, compassionate, and person-centred palliative care is qualitative data obtained through personal accounts and interviews with patients receiving palliative care. Notable are the accounts obtained during the review of the palliative care pathway the Liverpool Care Pathway in 2013 that illustrated that the pathway was no longer effective (Department of Health and Social Care, 2013). Without this vital, first-hand information, nurses, caregivers and other health and social care professionals would be relying on assumptions of how it feels to experience the complexity of mortality. Evidence to support necessary positive change would be left unsaid. Although every person and their situation and experience is different, without information obtained through qualitative research, nurses may find it more difficult to separate their personal views, morals and biases. This is necessary to remain objective and patient-centred when delivering palliative care.

Nurses bring their personal and professional experiences to their practice which contribute to the delivery of excellent care, which also evoke personal thoughts and feelings. This may compromise nurses' ability to separate their personal views from the patient's wishes, particularly in times of emotional intensity, such as supporting someone at the end of their life. This can be particularly challenging to navigate as a student when experiencing such situations for the first time.

A study by Westwood and Brown (2019) of student nurses at the University of Derby highlighted that over 72% had been exposed to a dying patient in their first placement. Almost 78% of the students felt that the education they received from their university course, up to that point, had not prepared them for this experience. This could be a factor as why Rachel is struggling to understand Fatima's choices regarding her care. Quantitative and qualitative research is important to gain evidence of student experiences as well as patients, all informing the best possible patient care. In Rachel and Ashely's situation, the Collaborative Learning in Practice (CliP) model encourages Ashley to support Rachel in navigating the challenges she is experiencing in delivering palliative care to Fatima. This support, through peer learning, has been shown to be an effective model of teaching for nursing students (Hill et al., 2020). Such experiences enhance learning and preparation for end-of-life care, delivered by university education teams. Both practice and education teams need to place research evidence at the centre of nursing practice and education with a commitment to patient and public involvement making this possible.

Patient and Public Involvement Pillar

The scenario outlined connects with patient and public involvement in many ways, with the sensitive nature of the case highlighting the need for nurses to listen to the patient voice. The importance of building a therapeutic relationship allows Ashley and the doctor mentioned, to advocate for Fatima's desires in line with the International Council of Nurses (2021) code. In Fatima's case, this involves ensuring she is treated as an individual and in a dignified manner and not making assumptions about her, particularly in relation to her faith and sexuality. Listening to Fatima allows for an understanding of her social and cultural background, which played a pivotal role in the decision-making process surrounding her care. Social and cultural awareness is crucial in the provision of holistic care (Mills, 2017).

By valuing the patient's voice, many aspects of this scenario are unveiled. Without active listening (for example, being attentive, understanding what is being said and responding meaningfully), Fatima's views around her care would not have been explored. Also, open conversations about her understanding of Ashley being non-binary would not have been had. This could have been detrimental to the care Fatima received as her wishes may not have been met. Efficient communication at the end of life is key to preventing misunderstandings and avoiding unnecessary distress (National Institute for Health and Care Excellence, 2023).

There is a delicate balance to be struck between recognising and respecting a patient's views, ideals, values and that of those providing care. In this scenario Fatima's right to be cared for by female staff becomes a complex issue when working with Ashley. Fatima's view that Ashley is male causes a dilemma when allocating staffing. As Ashley identifies as non-binary, this raises the question as to who can decide who provides care. It can be argued that a patient has the right to decline care provided by an individual and to request a different care-giver. In this scenario, by involving Fatima in a conversation without judgement, Rachel is attempting to advocate for Ashley while also respecting Fatima's right to decline care from Ashley. Fatima is placed at the centre of her care and the whole principle 'nothing about us, without us' (Charlton, 2000), as discussed in the PPI chapter, can be honoured.

Rachel and Ashley could have used this opportunity to speak to Fatima about her wishes, specifically why she declined any further treatment. This would allow Fatima to share her own narrative, in her own words, which can be a helpful form of expression and may encourage acceptance of Fatima's decisions as well as being educational for the students involved (Baines, Denniston, and Munro, 2019). As Sjögren Forss, Persson, and Borglin, (2019) explore, there is a significant shortfall in student nurse education when it comes to experiencing and understanding cultural diversity. This is where the PPI pillar can assist. Embedding a robust and effective PPI element into undergraduate nurse education, students can be better prepared and knowledgeable in providing care and support for patients like Fatima and her partner and family.

Engaging seriously with the integration of physical and mental health is the focus of the next pillar, which illuminates additional aspects of care scenario which are too often overlooked.

No Health without Mental Health Pillar

The scenario within this chapter allows for a complex appraisal of no health without mental health pillar. It is appropriate to consider mental health and well-being of both the patient, Fatima, and student nurses and this will be discussed in this section.

First, the patient's mental wellbeing must be addressed. Fatima has taken the decision to stop active treatment and has opted for palliative care. She is also distressed by the difficulties, likely to arise in her devout family, as a result of her relationship with Yumi. She is currently struggling with the decision as to how, or whether, to tell her parents and this could impact on her decision-making. Etengoff and Rodriguez (2021) report that many Muslim women, in same sex relationships, fear or are rejected by their families and have greater levels of depression as a result.

It is also important to consider how Fatima's physical health impacts on her mental health. Her cancer diagnosis, prognosis, and decision to follow the palliative care pathway will also affect her mental health. Greer et al. (2020) discuss how palliative care impacts on both patients' and caregivers' ability to cope. Fatima's decision will impact also her partner, Yumi. The progression of the cancer makes it likely that Fatima will require Yumi's help and support, intensifying as symptoms increase. This can put strain on a relationship and, in some instances, can lead to its breakdown (Greer et al., 2020). Fatima has the added complexity of her faith and family being potentially unsupportive of her relationship with Yumi. This could add further tensions within the relationship. Brent et al. (2018) explain the importance of family and friends' relationships throughout palliative care. A collaborative approach, taking into account both physical and mental health of Fatima and her family/support network is vital throughout the palliative care pathway. It is important that Rachel and Ashley support Fatima to ensure her mental health is considered as well as her physical health. Rachel and Ashley should not make assumptions about Fatima's mental health needs abut instead discuss these with her and look to offer mental health support both to Fatima and Yumi.

The second aspect to address is that of the mental health and well-being of the student nurses in this scenario. Providing care to patients with complex health needs, such as Fatima, can have a significant impact on nurses. Student nurses are, for example, especially susceptible to moral distress (Sasso et al., 2016). This is a particular challenge for Rachel as she struggles to comprehend Fatima's decision to take the palliative care pathway when there are treatment options. Rachel has knowledge that treatments are available that could prolong, and potentially improve, Fatima's quality of life. However, her decision not to take these options could result in Rachel feeling that she is not providing acceptable care which could impact on her mental health and well-being (Mæland et al., 2021).

Finally, the situation may also impact on Ashley's mental health and well-being. Ashley has experienced being 'misgendered' and, as Matsuno et al. (2022) argue, this is likely to be a common experience for Ashley. This can lead to feelings of invalidation and unacceptance and, ultimately, to poor mental health. Ashley has the added stressor of potentially having to explain their identify multiple times a day and potentially facing hostility, rejection or even aggression (Matsuno et al., 2022). Rachel, in this scenario, is an ally for Ashley, in advocating for them and attempting to support and educate others (see Chapter 1). Effective allies can improve psychological safety for individuals. A quarter of all student nurse will drop out before qualifying and the Royal College of Nursing attributes this to several reasons, including poor experiences in clinical practice (Perry, 2019). It is important therefore that student nurses look after their mental wellbeing and feel empowered and supported during clinical placements.

Nurses are needed to deliver excellence in health and social care. To do this well, they need to be attentive to equal consideration of physical and mental health. Without nurses sensitive to this, patients' interests and well-being will be compromised. Supporting and improving student and registered nurses' physical and mental health is as important as supporting them academically and practically. Caring for those who deliver care enhances their abilities to support the physical and mental health of the patients they care for.

The important role played by mental health nurses in responding globally has recently been recognised by the International Council of Nurses (2022). We discuss the global health pillar next.

Global Health Pillar

Breast cancer is the most common cancer diagnosis and leading cause of cancer-related death among females (0.5–1% of cases are men) (World Health Organization, 2021). Approximately half a million people die annually from metastatic breast cancer (Ahmad, 2019). Metastatic breast cancer is the most advanced form and is the costliest per person. The prevalence of metastatic breast cancer is expected to increase significantly over the next 10 years, with a greater proportion of younger people being diagnosed and care and treatment costs increasing by 140% (Gogate et al., 2021). There is also the emotional cost to the patient and their families, many struggle with the diagnosis and implications of it (Reed et al., 2012).

The prevalence of metastatic breast cancer varies across countries, and within individual countries, depending on the economic status, social and lifestyle factors relating to patients and diagnosis and the treatment infrastructure available. Western countries have the highest prevalence, with Asian and African countries having lower rates of early or primary breast cancer, however this is flipped for metastatic breast cancer. This is potentially due to the lack of infrastructure, and the economic status of the country and individuals (Bray et al., 2018). Ziegler et al. (1993) identified that, in low income migrating populations, incidence increased through the generations to that of the countries they moved to.

This shows how environmental, social, and economic factors impact on populations' risk. In high income countries fewer than 8% of patients are initially diagnosed with metastatic disease, in low-middle income countries 20–30% are initially diagnosed as metastatic (Unger-Saldaña, 2014). Access to innovative treatments, ongoing support and palliative care is also limited for those diagnosed. This is, in part, due to limited care coordination because of poor referral services. Progress and development requires collaboration between stakeholders to address these inequalities and unmet needs (Thrift-Perry et al., 2018).

Following the report on metastatic breast cancer by Cardoso et al. (2018), the Advanced Breast Cancer (ABC) Global Alliance was formed. The alliance works on common projects related to advanced breast cancer around the world. Their focus is to develop, promote and support awareness and actions that will improve and extend the lives of patients living with ABC worldwide. As a result, they developed the advanced breast cancer global charter. The charter lays out ten areas of focus to improve advanced breast cancer care. These include support patients to live longer, enhancing understanding of advanced breast cancer, improving the quality of life for patients, ensuring care is affordable and ensuring adequate communication for patients and between healthcare professionals.

Ashley and Rachel will continue to meet patients like Fatima, with diverse and complex needs, throughout their nursing careers. They need to ensure they have an awareness of the risks patients have of being diagnosed with common cancers and what the treatment options are. As student nurses, having an awareness of global health aspects of conditions such as breast cancer, is important. As discussed, those migrating from lower prevalence areas increase their individual risk the longer, they remain in high prevalence areas. Ashley and Rachel have a duty to ensure they provide education into risk factors and how to improve overall health, while also being aware of potential difficulties for patients to achieve this. Leadership – and management – are core capabilities for nurses to influence change at local and global levels. This is the final pillar explored in this chapter.

Leadership and Management Pillar

The leadership and management pillar of learning is of most importance when discussing Rachel and Ashley's approach to the collaborative provision of care. Strong leaders are vital in the navigation of ever evolving health and social care situations. In a multi-professional team, each professional brings experience and expertise to the care of patients, families and communities. Student professionals, also, bring a wealth of experience and should be supported and enabled to lead by example and deliver excellent care and to inspire those around to do the same.

Fatima's scenario provides opportunities for reflection on leadership and support between students. No leadership style is the same and most of the leaders of the present day manifest mixed leadership styles. Democratic leadership is often seen in Collaborative Learning in Practice model (CLIP) (Hill et al., 2020) environments, where more experienced students are leading and directing activities with less experienced students. The latter can seek guidance from the more experienced colleagues as needed. As Scheidlinger (1994) concluded, democratic working is favourable, intriguing, and enjoyable. As good as it may be for the learning environment, unfortunately, democratic styles are not as common in the 'real nursing world' due to influx of patients with complex needs. This leads to emergency situations that require a more authoritarian leadership style (Sfantou et al., 2017).

Self-discovery drives the sort of leader one may be and this stems from constant self-reflection. At the core of the practice of any registerd or student nurse are the aforementioned International Council of Nurses (2021) and Nursing and Midwifery Council (2018) codes. Therefore, for optimal learning of managerial skills to take place, nursing students alike Ashley and Rachel should have a clinical exposure experience to facilitate these learning opportunities. As per International Council of Nurses (2021), it is the nurse's role to educate their fellow colleagues about 'socio-political and economic issues that affect health including gender, ethnicity, race, culture, inequality and discrimination'.

Ashley, as a final year student, has developed significant clinical and interpersonal skills by this point on their learning journey., Therefore, encouraging Rachel to engage in focused reflection, with the Nursing and Midwifery Council (2018) Code in mind, would facilitate learning and self-awareness. Part 9.4 of the Code, 'support students' and colleagues' learning to help them develop their professional competence and confidence, is vital in the development of good leadership and management skills. Although, students are not bound by the code of practice until registration, their proficiencies are in accord with the Code and are crucial on completion of a programme.

Clinical placement areas are challenging settings to create an affirmative environment for first year students, like Rachel, due to rapid exposure to challenging dilemmas of nursing (Weurlander et al., 2018). The CLIP model (Hill, Woodward and Arthur, 2020) was developed to aid pre-registration nurses to learn from the experience of more senior students and encourages active peer learning and support in this challenging environment. The results of the Hill et al. (2020) study on the effectiveness of the CLIP Model in clinical practice, demonstrated a positive outcome in a lower total of students requiring learning plans, compared with those without the CLIP experience. It would be right to conclude that Ashley and Rachel are in a positive environment to apply the CLIP model and are greatly benefiting from student led learning.

Providing opportunities for students, like Ashley, to develop their leadership and management skills, are crucial prior to registration. This also applies to Rachel as guidance and role modelling are also crucial at the early stages of nurse education programmes. In addition, as the study results state, clinical areas should ensure that enough students of various stages are allocated to clinical area for the CLIP model to create the best possible learning and development environment (Hill et al., 2020).

Conclusion

This chapter, planned and authored by student nurses, created the opportunity to demonstrate collaborative learning and leadership in the integration of the seven pillars of learning to a complex care scenario. The complexity of nursing means that every patient and every interaction allows for in-depth, meaningful care. Also demonstrated is how student nurses can utilise and apply each pillar to develop their own nursing skills and ensure that patients receive high quality individualised care. In writing this chapter, student authors developed their own understanding of how the pillars apply in different ways to a single scenario. They have broken down the scenario to be able to better understand the potential difficulties that may occur and, therefore, plan ahead to manage and support everyone involved. In writing this chapter, students have shown how they can lead on care effectively and safely and are able to take this forward in their future practice. They will be able to utilise the skills, knowledge and values developed to support and educate both patients and other healthcare professionals as they develop in their nursing careers.

Takeaways for Student Nurses

- There is complexity within every patient interaction.
- Holistic care relies upon exceptional communication to enable a therapeutic dialogue between all participants.
- Application of all seven pillars enables effective, safe and ethical patient-centred care.
- Every interaction with patients, families and other healthcare professionals is a learning opportunity.
- Learning never stops and can come from a vast array of sources.

Takeaways for Educators/Practitioners

- The seven pillars give a structured approach to learning, providing guidance when attempting to break down complex scenarios.
- Allowing students to work using the pillars encourages interprofessional learning, a greater understanding of the wider impacts on healthcare provision and develops a sense of responsibility for students.

- Students are capable of understanding and recognising the complexities of care from early on within a pre-registration programme and allowing them to use and develop their curiosity encourages personal growth as well as professional development.
- Hierarchy in education is not always conducive to effective learning. All can learn from each other. An open approach allows for innovation, creativity and overall improved experiences for all.

References

Advanced Breast Cancer Global Alliance ESO initiative. (2017) 'ABC global charter 2017'. Available at: www.abcglobalalliance.org/wp-content/uploads/2018/01/ABC-Global-Charter-Booklet-Dec-2017.pdf (Accessed 18 April 2023).

Ahmad, A. (2019) 'Breast cancer statistics: Recent trends', in A. Ahmad (ed.), *Breast Cancer Metastasis and Drug Resistance Challenges and Progress*, 2nd edition. Available at: https://link.springer.com/book/10.1007/978-3-030-20301-6 (Accessed: 29 April 2023).

Baines, R., Denniston, C. and Munro, J. (2019) 'The transformative power of patient's narratives in healthcare education'. Available at: https://blogs.bmj.com/bmj/2019/07/08/the-transformative-power-of-patient-narratives-in-healthcare-education/#:~:text=For%20example%2C%20patient%20narratives%20can,professional%20identities%2C%20promote%20creativity%2C%20reinforce (Accessed: 18 April 2023).

Batstone, E. and Bailey, C. (2019) 'Spiritual care provision to end-of-life patients: A systematic literature review', *Journal of Clinical Nursing*, 29(19–20), pp. 3609–3642.

Beauchamp, T.L. and Childress, J.F. (2019) *Principles of Biomedical Ethics*, 8th edition. New York: Oxford University Press.

Bray, F., Ferlay, J., Soerjomataram, I., Siegel, R. L., Torre, L. A. and Jemal, A. (2018) 'Global cancer statistics 2018: GLOBOCAN estimates of incidence and mortality worldwide for 36 cancers in 185 countries;, *CA: A Cancer Journal for Clinicians*, 68, pp. 394–424.

Brent, L., Santy-Tomlinson, J. and Hertz, K. (2018) 'Family partnerships, palliative care and end of life', in L. Hertz, J. Santy-Tomlinson J. (eds), *Fragility Fracture Nursing: Holistic Care and Management of the Orthogeriatric Patient*. Available at: https://link.springer.com/book/10.1007/978-3-319-76681-2 (Accessed 21 April 2023).

Cardoso, F., Spence, D., Mertz, S., Corneliussen-James, D., Sabelko, K., Gralow, J., Cardoso, M.J., Peccatori, F., Paonessa, D., Benares, A., Sakurai, N., Beishon, M., Barker, S.-J. and Mayer, M. (2018) 'Global analysis of advanced/metastatic breast cancer: Decade report (2005–2015)', *The Breast*, 39, pp. 131–138.

Charlton, J. I. (2000) *Nothing about us without us: Disability Oppression and Empowerment*. California: University of California Press.

Department of Health and Social care. (2013) 'Independent report. Review of Liverpool Care Pathway for dying patients'. Available at: https://assets.publishing.service.gov.uk/government/uploads/system/uploads/attachment_data/file/212450/Liverpool_Care_Pathway.pdf (Accessed on 12 April 2023).

Etengoff, C. M. and Rodriguez, E.M. (2021) '"I feel as if I'm lying to them": Exploring Lesbian Muslims' Experiences of Rejection, Support, and Depression', *Journal of Homosexuality*, 68(7), pp. 1169–1195.

Fowler, M.D. (2021) 'Toward reclaiming our ethical heritage: Nursing ethics before bioethics', *The Online Journal of Issues in Nursing*, 25(04), pp. 1–4. Available at: www.proquest.com/openview/e5dcf37c1d78be7446d666b01716ac53/1?pq-origsite=gscholar&cbl=43860 (Accessed: 29 April 2023).

Gallagher, A. (2020) *Slow Ethics and the Art of Care*. Bradford: Emerald Publishing.

Gogate, A., Wheeler, S.B., Reeder-Hayes, K.E., Ekwueme, D.U., Fairley, T.L., Drier, S. and Trogdon, J.G. (2021) 'Projecting the prevalence and costs of metastatic breast cancer from 2015 through 2030', *JNCI Cancer Spectr.* 5(4), pp. 1–8.

Greer, J. A., Applebaum, A. J., Jacobsen, J. C., Temel, J. S. and Jackson, V. A. (2020) 'Understanding and addressing the role of coping in palliative care for patients with advanced cancer', *Journal of clinical oncology*, 38(9), pp. 915–925.

Hill, R., Woodward, M. and Arthur, A. (2020) 'Collaborative learning in practice (CLIP): Evaluation of a new approach to clinical learning', *Nurse Education Today*, 85, pp. 1–9.

Hunter-Jones, P., Sudbury-Riley, L., Al-Abdin, A. and Spence, C. (2022) 'The contribution of hospitality services to person-centred care: A study of the palliative care service ecosystem', *International Journal of Hospitality Management*, 103424, pp. 1–9.

International Council of Nurses. (2021) 'The ICN code of ethics for nurses'. Available at: www.icn.ch/system/files/2021-10/ICN_Code-of-Ethics_EN_Web_0.pdf (Accessed 24 April 2023).

International Council of Nurses (2022) 'The Global Mental Health Nursing Workforce: Time to prioritize and invest in mental health and wellbeing'. Available at: www.icn.ch/sites/default/files/inline-files/ICN_Mental_Health_Workforce_report_EN_web.pdf [Accessed 7 July 2023].

Kitson, A, Athlin, A. and Conroy, T. (2014) 'Anything but basic: Nursing's challenge in meeting patients fundamental care needs', *Journal of Nursing Scholarship*, 46(5), pp. 331–339.

Mæland, M. K., Tingvatn, B. S., Rykkje, L. and Drageset, S. (2021) 'Nursing education: Students' narratives of moral distress in clinical practice', *Nursing Reports*, 11(2), pp. 291–300.

Matsuno, E., Bricker, N. L., Savarese, E., Mohr, R., Jr. and Balsam, K. F. (2022) '"The default is just going to be getting misgendered": Minority stress experiences among nonbinary adults', *Psychology of Sexual Orientation and Gender Diversity*', Advance online publication, pp. 1–13.

Mills, I.J. (2017) 'A person-centred approach to holistic assessment', *Primary Dental Journal*, 6(3), pp. 18–23.

Musto, L. C., Rodney, P.A. and Vanderheide, R. (2015) 'Toward interventions to address moral distress: navigating structure and agency', *Nursing Ethics*, 22(1), pp. 91–102.

National Institute for Health and Care Excellence. (2020a) 'Impact of end of life care for adults'. Available at: www.nice.org.uk/about/what-we-do/into-practice/measuring-the-use-of-nice-guidance/impact-of-our-guidance/nice-impact-end-of-life-care-for-adults (Accessed: 17 April 2023).

National Institute for Health and Care Excellence. (2023) 'Shared decision making'. Available at: www.nice.org.uk/about/what-we-do/our-programmes/nice-guidance/nice-guidelines/shared-decision-making (Accessed 17 April 2023).

Nursing and Midwifery Council. (2018) 'The Code. Professional standards of practice and behaviour for nurses and midwives'. Available at: www.nmc.org.uk/standards/code/ (Accessed: 9 January 2023).

Pedersen, B. and Sivonen, K. (2012) 'The impact of clinical encounters on student nurses' ethical caring', *Nursing Ethics*, 19(6) pp. 838–848.

Perry, S. (2019) 'Nursing students are still dropping out in worrying numbers'. Available at: www.health.org.uk/news-and-comment/news/a-quarter-of-all-nursing-students-are-dropping-out-of-their-degrees (Accessed: 18 April 2023).

Reed, E., Simmonds, P., Haviland, J. and Corner, J. (2012) 'Quality of life and experience of care in women with metastatic breast cancer: A cross-sectional survey', *Journal of Pain and Symptom Management*, 43(4), pp. 747–758.

Roach, S. (2002) *Caring, the Human Mode of Being: A Blueprint for the Health Professions*, 2nd edition. Ottawa: CHA Press.

Sasso, L., Bagnasco, A., Bianchi, M., Bressan, V. and Carnevale, F. (2016) 'Moral distress in undergraduate nursing students: A systematic review', *Nursing Ethics*, 23(5), pp. 523–534.

Scheidlinger, S. (1994) 'The Lewin, Lippitt and White study of leadership and "social climates" revisited', *International Journal of Group Psychotherapy*, 44(1), pp. 123–127.

Selman, L., Speck, P., Barfield, R. C., Gysels, M., Higginson, I. J. and Harding, R. (2014) 'Holistic models for end of life care: Establishing the place of culture', *Progress in Palliative Care*, 22(2), pp. 80–87.

Sfantou, D., Laliotis, A., Patelarou, A.E., Sifaki-Pistolla, D., Matalliotakis, M. And Patelarou, E.(2017) 'Importance of leadership style towards quality of care measures in healthcare settings: A systematic review', *Healthcare*, 5(4), pp. 1–17.

Sjögren Forss, K., Persson, K. and Borglin, G. (2019) 'Nursing students' experiences of caring for ethnically and culturally diverse patients. A scoping review', *Nurse Education in Practice*, 37, pp. 97–104.

Thrift-Perry, M., Cabanes, A., Cardoso, F., Hunt, K.M., Cruz, T.A. and Faircloth, K. (2018) 'Global analysis of metastatic breast cancer policy gaps and advocacy efforts across the patient journey', *The Breast*, 41, pp. 93–106.

Unger-Saldaña, K. (2014) 'Challenges to the early diagnosis and treatment of breast cancer in developing countries', *World Journal of Clinical Oncology*, 5(3), pp. 465–477.

Westwood, S. and Brown, M. (2019) Preparing students to care for patients at the end of life. *Nursing Times*, 115(10) pp. 43–46.

Weurlander, M., Lonn, A., Seeberger, A., Broberger, E., Hult, H. and Wernerson, A. (2018) 'How do medical and nursing students experience emotional challenges during clinical placements?' *International Journal of Medical Education*, 9, pp. 74–82.

Wolf, Z.R. and Langer, S. (2000) 'The meaning of nursing practice in the stories and poems of nurses working in hospitals: a phenomenological study', *Journal of Human Caring*, 4(3), pp. 7–17.

World Health Organization (2020) *Basic Documents*, 49th Edition. Available at: https://apps.who.int/gb/bd/pdf_files/BD_49th-en.pdf [Accessed: July 7th 2023].

World Health Organization. (2021) 'Breast cancer'. Available at: www.who.int/news-room/fact-sheets/detail/breast-cancer (Accessed 24 April 2023).

Ziegler, R.G., Hoover, R.N., Pike, M.C., Hildesheim, A., Nomura, A.M.Y., West, D.W., Wu-Williams, A.H., Kolonel, L.N., Horn-Ross, P.L., Rosenthal, J.F. and Hyer, M.B. (1993) 'Migration patterns and breast cancer risk in Asian-American women', *JNCI: Journal of the National Cancer Institute*, 85(22), pp. 1819–1827.

10 Conclusion
Context and Reflective Questions

Ann Gallagher

Introduction

In writing this concluding section of our co-produced book, it is appropriate to reflect on the journey to completion. A journey which has foregrounded the value of co-production with a diverse group of authors with a common purpose: to contribute to the betterment of nursing practice and education through scholarship. It is our view that the seven pillars of learning, explored in this book, are necessary components of the aspiration to excellence in health and social care. However, we accept they may not be sufficient, and others may be added to enhance nursing curricula in other cultural contexts and in response to future developments in care practices, locally and globally.

Context

As outgoing head of nursing at the University of Exeter, I am mindful of the significance of closing chapters – and opening others – for some of our student authors and for myself. Our final-year students, pioneers of the Exeter MSci Nursing Programme, are soon to graduate and become registered nurses. They have had a challenging and interesting student journey as they negotiated the impact of the COVID-19 pandemic and experienced the pleasures and the pain of the first run of a new nurse education programme. Exeter students' resilience, tenacity, and commitment to excellence in care have been inspiring and this book will be part of their legacy to future cohorts of student nurses everywhere.

As discussed in Chapter 1, our book was developed during a period of increasing complexity and challenges impacting nursing. As I write these concluding comments, media attention continues to focus on nurses' strikes in England, to individual and organisational failures in public services, to conflict in Ukraine and in Sudan and to the environmental crisis. There is also increasing attention to the benefits and risks of artificial intelligence (AI), particularly in relation to education. The creation of tools such as ChatGPT, for example, introduces challenges which impact nursing practice and education directly (Lateef Alkhaqani, 2023).

The launch of a report on *The Future of Ageing* (Nuffield Council on Bioethics, 2023), which I attended as a working group member, coincided with the completion of our book. The report explored the potential impact of biomedical and technological developments to enhance later years. This report – and discussions around it – have much relevance to nursing practice and education as we respond to an ageing population with escalating care needs.

DOI: 10.4324/9781003390565-10

The collaborative effort in co-producing this text would not have been possible without the generosity, patience and dedication of every one of the 36 contributors. The expertise and experience of students, PPI members and the Academy of Nursing team have been willingly shared and have creatively integrated theory and practice. It has been a privilege to work with all of these committed authors and to learn from their insights, particularly in the sharing, refinement and analysis of the anonymised scenarios. The relevance and value of the seven pillars of learning are demonstrated by application to these practice scenarios. The scenarios enabled chapter authors to apply wide-ranging knowledge, skills and values relating to the pillars. The scenarios are short stories which are intended to engage and prompt readers' towards an enhanced understanding of nursing practice and education. As Arthur Frank (2010, p. 3) writes:

> Stories animate human life; that is their work. Stories work with people, for people and always stories work on people. Stories affect what people are able to see as real, as possible, and as worth doing or best avoided.

The stories and chapters also illustrate ways in which curiosity, advocacy, respect, and excellence – the book's CARE themes – are threaded through the pillar chapters.

Reflective Questions: The Seven Pillars of Learning

This chapter is intended as consolidation and as providing a range of reflective questions to deepen students' learning. It is also intended that they serve as a resource for educators and practitioners to stimulate critical discussion regarding the application of the seven pillars to nursing practice.

Readers may recall, from our introduction, the statement that 'each academic field can be *defined* by its essential questions' (Eyler, 2018, p. 43). There, we suggested some broad questions regarding the meaning of the 'good nurse' and consideration of the factors that enhance or challenge the development of the profession. Here we suggest a range of questions which are designed to be helpful as a self-assessment of readers' own understanding of the seven pillars and also to facilitate group discussions.

1. Fundamentals of Nursing Care Pillar

- What is meant by the fundamentals of care?
- How would you recognise nursing practice which prioritises fundamentals of care?
- What difference does the enactment of fundamentals of care pillar make to the experiences of patients and families? Share three examples.

2. Ethics and Professionalism Pillar

- What do you understand by ethics in relation to nursing practice?
- How would you explain professionalism to a first-year student nurse?
- When have you witnessed ethics and professionalism demonstrated in health or social care?
- What difference does the enactment of the ethics and professionalism pillar to the experience of patients and families? Share three examples.

3. *Evidence for Nursing Practice Pillar*

- What do you understand by evidence in relation to nursing practice?
- How have you applied evidence to your nursing practice? Give 3 examples.
- What difference has the application of the evidence in practice pillar made to the experience of patients and families? Share three examples.

4. *Patient and Public Involvement Pillar*

- What does Patient and Public Involvement mean?
- Why is it important in nurse education? Suggest 3 examples.
- What difference does the involvement of PPI group members make to student nurses? Share three examples from nurse education.

5. *No Health without Mental Health Pillar*

- What do you understand by No Health without Mental Health?
- In what practice circumstances have you witnessed the application of this pillar?
- What difference does the application of the No Health Without Mental Health Pillar make to the experience of patients and families? Share three examples.

6. *Global Health Pillar*

- What does global health mean?
- How does the global health pillar impact nursing practice in your cultural context?
- What difference does an understanding of the global health pillar make to patients and families? Provide three examples.

7. *Leadership and Management Pillar*

- What do you think is the difference between management and leadership in nursing practice? Give examples to illustrate.
- Reflecting on your own role in nursing practice and education, in what situations are you acting as a manager? And when are you acting as a leader?
- When have you witnessed nurse leadership making a difference to patients and families? Share three examples.

Additional Pillars of Learning?

- Reflect on your own practice and consider if there are additional pillars you think should be added to those explored in this book?
- Discuss your arguments for the additional pillar(s) – if any – with other student nurses and educators.

Reflective Questions Relating to CARE

In Chapter 1 we introduced the CARE themes, which are threaded through the book. In this section, we suggest some hypothetical situations intended to stimulate reflection on the implications of these themes for nursing practice and education.

Curiosity

- Imagine a student nurse who lacks curiosity. Discuss with a friend or colleague how this student would interact with a patient? With the patient's family? With a colleague?
- Consider now, a student nurse who is overly curious, asking many questions of patients and families. How, do you think, would this be received? What guidance might you provide to such students regarding the right amount of curiosity in professional practice? Which questions are acceptable? Which are not?
- Share an example of an experienced nurse you have worked with, who demonstrates curiosity in an effective and ethical manner.

Advocacy

- Imagine a student nurse who lacks knowledge of, and skills relating to, patient advocacy and allyship. How is this lack of competence and commitment likely to impact the student's relationship with patients? Families? And colleagues?
- Consider now, a student nurse who takes the role of advocate seriously and who takes it on themselves to speak up for patients at every opportunity. What might the consequences be of this approach to patient advocacy? What guidance might you give to this student regarding appropriate patient advocacy?
- Share an example of an experienced nurse you have worked with, who demonstrates patient advocacy in an appropriate and ethical manner.

Respect

- Imagine a student nurse who is disrespectful towards a patient or colleague. Consider the ways the student could be disrespectful? What behaviours and attitudes might they demonstrate?
- Consider now, a student who appears overly respectful to patients and colleagues. How might they appear? What behaviours and attitudes might they demonstrate? How might you advise this student as to how they balance self-respect and respect for others?
- Share an example of an experienced nurse you have worked with, who demonstrates respect in an effective and ethical manner.

Excellence

- Imagine a situation where a student nurse challenges the idea of excellence in health and social care. They tell you this is impossible and pointless. Nurses should be content to deliver minimal care given short-staffing and the crisis in health services. How would you respond to this student?
- Consider now, a student who tells you they are unable to continue on their nurse education programme because they feel they are always cutting corners and not delivering good care. How might you advise this student regarding the role of nurses in aspiring to excellence in care?
- Share an example of an experienced nurse you have worked with, who demonstrates an aspiration to excellence in health and/or social care.

Conclusion

It is intended that the seven pillars of learning will engage and inspire readers and also strengthen their commitment to develop and advance the profession of nursing. It is hoped that readers will better appreciate their critical role in supporting the flourishing of patients, families and communities and also their own flourishing as exemplary nurse leaders. It is also hoped also, as expressed in the introduction, that students' confidence and competence gained from working through this book will inspire and strengthen their aspiration to excellence in health and social care.

It has been a pleasure working with my co-editors, Kris Deering and Enrico De Luca, and with Exeter student nurses, the Academy of Nursing patient and public involvement (PPI) group, and the nurse education team. This book signals a celebration of what can be achieved when there is a successful collaboration of people who care about nursing and who are committed to making a positive difference to the lives of patients, families, and communities. People with a shared common purpose in solidarity with each other. It is hoped that our co-production process, characterised by reflection, respect and dialogue with each other, be replicated by nurse leaders in practice, education and research everywhere.

References

Alkhaqani, A.L. (2023) 'ChatGPT and Nursing Education: Challenges and Opportunities', *Journal of Medical Science*, 4, pp. 50–51. Available at: www.researchgate.net/publication/369625345_ChatGPT_and_Nursing_Education_Challenges_and_Opportunities (Accessed 28 April 2023).

Eyler, J.R. (2018) *How Humans Learn: The Science and Stories Behind Effective College Teaching.* Morgantown, WV: West Virginia University Press.

Frank, A. (2010) *Letting Stories Breathe: A Socio-narratology.* Chicago, IL: University of Chicago Press.

Nuffield Council on Bioethics. (2023) *The Future of Ageing: Ethical Considerations for Research and Innovation.* London: Nuffield Council on Bioethics.

Index

Entries in *italics* denote figures.

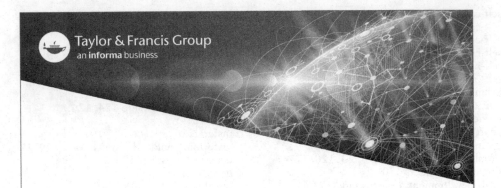

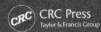